Health Policy and Advocacy in Hand Surgery

Editor

KEVIN C. CHUNG

HAND CLINICS

www.hand.theclinics.com

Consulting Editor
KEVIN C. CHUNG

May 2020 • Volume 36 • Number 2

ELSEVIER

1600 John F. Kennedy Boulevard • Suite 1800 • Philadelphia, Pennsylvania, 19103-2899

http://www.theclinics.com

HAND CLINICS Volume 36, Number 2
May 2020 ISSN 0749-0712, ISBN-13: 978-0-323-71338-2

Editor: Lauren Boyle
Developmental Editor: Kristen Helm

Hand Clinics (ISSN 0749-0712) is published quarterly by Elsevier Inc., 360 Park Avenue South, New York, NY 10010-1710. Months of publication are February, May, August, and November. Business and Editorial Offices: 1600 John F. Kennedy Blvd., Ste. 1800, Philadelphia, PA 19103-2899. Customer Service Office: 3251 Riverport Lane, Maryland Heights, MO 63043. Periodicals postage paid at New York, NY and at additional mailing offices. Subscription price is $439.00 per year (domestic individuals), $854.00 per year (domestic institutions), $100.00 per year (domestic students/residents), $501.00 per year (Canadian individuals), $994.00 per year (Canadian institutions), $562.00 per year (international individuals), $994.00 per year (international institutions), $256.00 (international students/residents), and $100.00 (Canadian students/residents). Foreign air speed delivery is included in all *Clinics* subscription prices. All prices are subject to change without notice. **POSTMASTER:** Send address changes to *Hand Clinics*, Elsevier Health Sciences Division, Subscription Customer Service, 3251 Riverport Lane, Maryland Heights, MO 63043. Customer Service (orders, claims, online, change of address): Elsevier Health Sciences Division, Subscription **Customer Service, 3251 Riverport Lane, Maryland Heights, MO 63043. Tel: 1-800-654-2452 (U.S. and Canada); 314-447-8871 (outside U.S. and Canada). Fax: 314-447-8029. E-mail: journalscustomerservice-usa@elsevier.com (for print support); journalsonlinesupport-usa@elsevier.com (for online support).**

Reprints. For copies of 100 or more of articles in this publication, please contact the Commercial Reprints Department, Elsevier Inc., 360 Park Avenue South, New York, New York 10010-1710. Tel.: 212-633-3874; Fax: 212-633-3820; E-mail: reprints@elsevier.com.

Hand Clinics is covered in *MEDLINE/PubMed (Index Medicus), Current Contents/Clinical Medicine, EMBASE/Excerpta Medica,* and *ISI/BIOMED.*

Contributors

CONSULTING EDITOR

KEVIN C. CHUNG, MD, MS
Charles B. G. de Nancrede Professor of
Surgery, Professor of Plastic Surgery and
Orthopaedic Surgery, Chief of Hand Surgery,
Michigan Medicine, Assistant Dean for Faculty
Affairs, Associate Director of Global REACH,
University of Michigan Medical School, Ann
Arbor, Michigan, USA

EDITOR

KEVIN C. CHUNG, MD, MS
Charles B. G. de Nancrede Professor of
Surgery, Professor of Plastic Surgery and
Orthopaedic Surgery, Chief of Hand Surgery,
Michigan Medicine, Assistant Dean for Faculty
Affairs, Associate Director of Global REACH,
University of Michigan Medical School, Ann
Arbor, Michigan, USA

AUTHORS

NATALIE B. BAXTER, BSE
Clinical Research Assistant, Section of Plastic
Surgery, Department of Surgery, University of
Michigan Medical School, Michigan Medicine,
Ann Arbor, Michigan, USA

CHRISTINA I. BRADY, MD
Assistant Professor, Department of
Orthopaedic Surgery, UT Health San Antonio,
San Antonio, Texas, USA

GREGORY D. BYRD, MD, MA
Olympia Orthopaedic Associates, Olympia,
Washington, USA

**DANIEL CADOUX-HUDSON, MRCS(Eng),
MBBS, BSc**
Specialist Registrar, Hand Unit, University
Hospital Southampton, Southampton,
United Kingdom

KEVIN C. CHUNG, MD, MS
Charles B. G. de Nancrede Professor of
Surgery, Professor of Plastic Surgery and
Orthopaedic Surgery, Chief of Hand Surgery,
Michigan Medicine, Assistant Dean for Faculty
Affairs, Associate Director of Global REACH,
University of Michigan Medical School, Ann
Arbor, Michigan, USA

CHRISTOPHER J. DY, MD, MPH, FACS
Assistant Professor, Department of
Orthopaedic Surgery, Washington University
School of Medicine, St Louis, Missouri, USA

ANDREW GURMAN, MD
Former President of the AMA, Solo Hand
Surgery Practice, Altoona, Pennsylvania, USA

KRISTINE A. HUYNH, BS
Medical Student, Oakland University William
Beaumont School of Medicine, Rochester,
Michigan, USA

ROBIN N. KAMAL, MD
Department of Orthopaedic Surgery, Stanford University, Redwood City, California, USA

ROBERT L. KANE, BS
Clinical Research Associate, Section of Plastic Surgery, Department of Surgery, University of Michigan Medical School, Ann Arbor, Michigan, USA

PREETHI KESAVAN, BS
Medical Student, Washington University School of Medicine, St Louis, Missouri, USA

LESLEY KHAN-FAROOQI, OTD, OTR, CHT
ASHT Practice Division Director, Assistant Professor, Occupational Therapy Program, University of St. Augustine, Austin, Texas, USA

KAY KIRKPATRICK, MD
Senator, Former President of Resurgens Orthopaedics, Georgia State Senate, Atlanta, Georgia, USA

JASMINE KRISHNAN, OTRL, CHT, MHSA, BSc(H)OT
Occupational Therapist, Certified Hand Therapist, Michigan Medicine, Rehabilitation Services, Domino's Farms, Ann Arbor, Michigan, USA

LARS MATKIN, MD, MBA
Orthopedic Surgery Department, The University of Texas at Austin, Austin, Texas, USA

WALTER B. McCLELLAND Jr, MD, FAAOS, FAOA
Peachtree Orthopedics, Atlanta, Georgia, USA

STEPHEN M. McCOLLAM, MD, FAAOS, FAOA
Peachtree Orthopedics, Atlanta, Georgia, USA

ANNE J. MILLER-BRESLOW, MD
Consultant, Englewood Hospital Medical Center, Englewood, New Jersey, USA

JACOB S. NASSER, BS
Medical Student, The George Washington School of Medicine & Health Sciences, Washington DC, USA

EKTA PATHARE, FACHE, MBA, OTR, CHT
President, CGAIT Global LLC, Vice Practice Division Director, ASHT, Vice Chair, Education Committee, ACHE of North Texas, Coppell, Texas, USA

NOAH M. RAIZMAN, MD, MFA
Assistant Clinical Professor, The George Washington University, Washington, DC, USA

DAVID RING, MD, PhD
Department of Surgery and Perioperative Care, The University of Texas at Austin, Austin, Texas, USA

JAMES M. SAUCEDO, MD, MBA
Orthopedics and Sports Medicine, Houston Methodist Hospital, Houston, Texas, USA

LAUREN M. SHAPIRO, MD
Department of Orthopaedic Surgery, Stanford University, Stanford, California, USA

LEE SQUITIERI, MD, PhD, MS
Resident Physician, Division of Plastic and Reconstructive Surgery, Department of Surgery, Keck School of Medicine of USC, University of Southern California, Los Angeles, California, USA

JENNIFER F. WALJEE, MD, MPH
Associate Professor of Surgery, Section of Plastic Surgery, Department of Surgery, Michigan Medicine, Ann Arbor, Michigan, USA

DAVID WARWICK, MD, FRCS (Orth)
European Diploma of Hand Surgery, Professor, Consultant Hand Surgeon, Hand Unit, University Hospital Southampton, Southampton, United Kingdom

DAVID WEI, MD, MS
Hand and Upper Extremity Surgeon, Orthopaedic and Neurosurgery Specialists, Greenwich, Connecticut, USA

ARNOLD-PETER C. WEISS, MD
R. Scot Sellers Scholar of Hand Surgery, Chief, Hand and Upper Extremity Surgery, Professor and Vice Chair, Department of Orthopaedics, The Warren Alpert Medical School of Brown University, Providence, Rhode Island, USA; University Orthopedics, East Providence, Rhode Island, USA

Contents

Collaboration with organizations beyond the clinical setting is necessary to identify safety hazards that contribute to the high incidence and severity of hand conditions. Hand surgeons are acutely aware of obstacles patients face while navigating the health care system. Advocacy efforts encourage the development of equitable insurance policies and improve health resource allocation so that hand surgeons can treat a larger patient population. Participation in quality initiatives supports the development of evidence-based clinical guidelines. Further evidence must be generated to ensure that surgeons remain proficient in the latest techniques and uphold high standards of care as hand surgery procedures evolve.

Despite the significant investment in scientific investigation to enhance clinical care, the uptake of new interventions and innovations into clinical care and policy remains slow. Understanding and examining the factors that influence the dissemination and implementation of best practices are critical to promote high-quality health care. This review provides an overview of the evidence base in hand surgery, the science that underlies dissemination and innovation, and the emergence of learning health systems in health care.

Each step of the evidence-based practice process is critical and requires clear understanding for accurate application. To practice evidence-based care, providers must acquire a specific skillset that facilitates translation of a patient problem into an answerable research question. Additional requirements are understanding of electronic databases, critical appraisal of the available evidence, and integration of the findings to generate a specific, individualized treatment plan. Although this process is demanding, evidence-based practice is essential in the delivery of optimal patient care.

Hand surgery researchers should focus on developing high-quality evidence to support the development of health policies affecting surgical care. Policy-makers and leaders of national hand societies can help reduce the variation of care for patients receiving hand surgery by incorporating evidence into guidelines and policies. Comprehensive guidelines for perioperative care help encourage the translation of evidence into practice. Moreover, the identification of institutional-level barriers and facilitators of integration ensures the successful implementation of hand surgery–specific programs. The development of robust metrics to evaluate the effect of policy on practice helps examine the feasibility of clinical guidelines.

centralized system that tracks process and outcome measures, delivers national benchmarking, and encourages the sharing of knowledge. A national registry can fulfill these needs for hand surgeons and incorporate quality improvement into their daily routine. Leaders in hand surgery should convene to appraise the organization of a national registry for their field and reach consensus on how the registry can be designed and funded.

Health services research using secondary data is a powerful tool for guiding quality/performance measure development, payment reform, and health policy. Patient preferences, physical examination findings, use of postoperative care, and other factors specific to hand surgery research are critical pieces of information required to study quality of care and improve patient outcomes. These data often are missing from data sets, causing limitations and challenges when performing secondary data analyses in hand surgery. As the role of secondary data in surgical research expands, hand surgeons must apply novel strategies and become involved in collaborative initiatives to overcome the limitations of existing resources.

Economically vulnerable US patients are at risk for undertreatment of hand-related conditions as well as poorer outcomes. The cost of indigent care can be substantial to both the patients and their communities. Caring for these patients in a system that depends on inconsistent coverage requires a network of safety-net hospitals. To ensure that patients have access to care, the protection of safety-net hospitals should be prioritized when discussing federal and state funding allocation. On an individual scale, surgeons can also make changes in their practices to help find sustainable ways to care for indigent patients.

The medical device industry has long been subject to criticism for lack of price transparency and minimal regulations surrounding device approval, which have functioned as barriers to providing quality and cost-effective care. Recent health care reforms aimed at overcoming these barriers, including improving market approval regulations, increasing postmarket surveillance, and using comparative effectiveness research, have drastically changed industry practices. These reforms have also prompted increasingly cost-aware health care practices, which have encouraged new trends in medical device innovation such as frugal innovation and deinstitutionalization. This article explores the challenges faced by industry, physicians, and patients in light of these reforms.

Health policy is a complex and fluid topic that addresses care delivery with the goal of improving patient care. Understanding health policy initiatives, their motivation, and their effects, can help ensure hand surgeons are prepared for the changing health care landscape.

Advocacy and the Hand Surgeon: Why and How   271

Kay Kirkpatrick and Andrew Gurman

This article explains and gives examples of the importance of political advocacy for hand surgeons at the federal and state levels. Two health care leaders who are also hand surgeons, one now serving as a state Senator and one a former President of the American Medical Association, give their perspective on participation in the political process. The article covers avenues for advocacy for hand surgeons as individuals and as members of medical organizations, including suggestions about effective communication with legislators. There is discussion of the unique role of the American Society for Surgery of the Hand in representing hand surgeons.

HAND CLINICS

SERIES OF RELATED INTEREST:

Clinics in Plastic Surgery
https://www.plasticsurgery.theclinics.com/

Orthopedic Clinics of North America
https://www.orthopedic.theclinics.com/

Physical Medicine and Rehabilitation Clinics of North America
https://www.pmr.theclinics.com/

THE CLINICS ARE AVAILABLE ONLINE!
Access your subscription at:
www.theclinics.com

Preface

Guiding the Future of Hand Surgery Through Health Policy and Advocacy

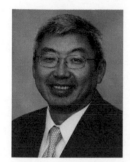

Kevin C. Chung, MD, MS
Editor

Health policy has become indispensable for the delivery of effective and equitable care in the complex, nuanced American health care system. This *Hand Clinics* issue describes how health care policy influences the practice of hand surgery across the outpatient and inpatient arenas. Surgeons have an evolving relationship with hospitals and continuously adapt to new regulations enacted by insurance companies and the government. We cannot ignore the calls for quality of care over quantity of care. Policymakers are insisting that physicians demonstrate the value of care not only to enhance health outcomes but also to lower costs.

We have assembled visionary leaders from hand surgery to share their insights on outcomes assessment, value-based care, the challenges of running a private practice, and the need for data collection through a national hand surgery registry. In addition, surgeons who have served on the leadership of the American Medical Association and state legislatures discuss how the political landscape is shaping the current and future delivery of health care. Practical, immediately applicable topics include the efficient use of electronic medical records, optimization of reimbursements, and partnership with industry. Our colleagues also provide a balanced observation of the British National Health Service in light of

the United States' possible transition toward universal health care. We should not ignore the uninsured and underinsured, who are the most vulnerable during any changes in policy. Furthermore, we should continue to cherish our relationship with our hand therapists, who adroitly provide their wisdom for this most essential need of our patients.

I am pleased to announce my presidential theme, as the 75th President of the American Society of Surgery of the Hand, is health policy and advocacy. During my Presidential year, I wish to leverage the guidance provided in this issue to shape the future of our specialty so that we can overcome many of the challenges that are upon us. Collectively, we in the hand surgery community strive to shape a better future for patients, our specialty, and our nation.

Kevin C. Chung, MD, MS
Michigan Medicine
1500 East Medical Center Drive
2130 Taubman Center, SPC 5340
Ann Arbor, MI 48109, USA

E-mail address:
kecchung@med.umich.edu

Hand Clin 36 (2020) xi
https://doi.org/10.1016/j.hcl.2020.02.001
0749-0712/20/© 2020 Published by Elsevier Inc.

Navigating the Intersection of Evidence and Policy in Hand Surgery Practice

Natalie B. Baxter, BSE[a], Kevin C. Chung, MD, MS[b],*

KEYWORDS

- Hand surgery • Health policy • Evidence-based medicine • Patient advocacy
- Access to health care • Quality of care

KEY POINTS

- Enactment of policy to address injury prevention and resource allocation in the emergency setting becomes increasingly important as the incidence of traumatic injuries rises.
- Hand surgeons' efforts to communicate health disparities to policymakers, in the form of qualitative and quantitative evidence, encourage health care reform that expands patient access to care.
- Quality measures are necessary to establish evidence-based practices and adapt to value-based insurance structures; however, tools unique to hand surgery are lacking.
- Participation in collaborative research and development of novel methods for analyses eases the integration of new technologies into practice.

Health research spending in the United States increased by 21% between 2013 and 2016 and now exceeds $170 billion per year.[1] Despite this enormous expenditure, the rationale for various health-related policies diverges from what the evidence proves is effective. Investigators argue that a lack of high-quality evidence makes it difficult to justify new policies.[2,3] Meanwhile others maintain that efforts are misplaced; the necessary evidence exists, but it is improperly conveyed to policymakers.[4] Both explanations assume that evidence and policy are directly and irreversibly linked. However, the creation of policy is a dynamic process, requiring quantitative and qualitative evidence from clinical investigations, public health research, and even narrative accounts. Although the influence of government-enacted laws and regulations is well recognized, the narrower impacts of clinical guidelines and internal agency decisions diffuse throughout the health care system.[5] Continued generation of evidence is necessary to assess the effectiveness of health policies and rapidly adapt to the evolving health care landscape.

Regardless of the motives or authority of the enforcing body, the impact of policy affects all levels of the health care system. Efforts to limit tobacco use, for example, took off in 1964 when the US Surgeon General reported on the severe health hazards of cigarette smoking.[6] This led to the enactment of federal and state policies that require warning labels on cigarette packaging and ban smoking in public places.[7] A concerted effort by the Agency for Healthcare Research and Quality and Centers for Disease Control and Prevention, among others, resulted in the establishment of clinical practice guidelines that health care professionals may use to promote smoking-cessation.[8]

[a] Section of Plastic Surgery, Department of Surgery, University of Michigan Medical School, Michigan Medicine, 1500 East Medical Center Drive, 2130 Taubman Center, Ann Arbor, MI 48109-5231, USA; [b] Section of Plastic Surgery, Michigan Medicine, 1500 East Medical Center Drive, 2130 Taubman Center, SPC 5340, Ann Arbor, MI 48109-5340, USA
* Corresponding author.
E-mail address: kecchung@med.umich.edu

Hand Clin 36 (2020) 123–129
https://doi.org/10.1016/j.hcl.2020.01.001
0749-0712/20/© 2020 Elsevier Inc. All rights reserved.

Although tobacco use remains a major public health issue, the US smoking rate has dropped by more than 50% over the last half-century following the execution of these initiatives.[6] Research indicates that smoking slows wound healing and worsens certain hand conditions. Thus, policies to curb tobacco use can have significant effects in hand surgery.[9]

Health policy is beneficial for individuals and society at large. However, the immediate impact of policy is often difficult to ascertain and may in fact be harmful. The opioid crisis has revealed the consequences that arise when clinical guidelines are misdirected or lack detail. Opioids are regularly prescribed after hand surgery, although guidelines rarely specify what quantifies a reasonable dose and few surgical training programs include pain management in their curricula.[10] As a result, the quantity of medication prescribed to patients varies widely. Johnson and colleagues[11] observed that 13% of opioid-naive patients continued to fill-prescriptions months after surgery. This number is concerning given that far fewer patients seem to experience postoperative complications that necessitate continued pain management. Although overprescription of opioids is prevalent in many areas of medicine, this information reinforces the need for well-supported, specialty-specific guidelines. Evidence and health policy are not connected by a one-way street. Constant evaluation and feedback ensures that policies address issues unique to hand surgery and facilitate progress within the specialty.

In this article we present a conceptual model to portray how evidence and policy give insight to the challenges faced by hand surgery patients and providers. Because the cause of injuries is wide-ranging, we first focus on the factors upstream of the clinical setting that introduce a need for hand surgery and obstruct access to health care. We then discuss discrepancies in quality of care and how best practices are defined. Finally, we consider how professionals within hand surgery can act to move the specialty forward.

CONCEPTUAL MODEL

We created a conceptual model to convey how evidence and policy influence hand surgery (**Fig. 1**). The elements of this model include (1) incidence of injury, (2) access to health care, (3) quality of care, and (4) innovation in hand surgery. Although the elements are presented separately, their impacts are not always distinct. A collection of evidence from multiple perspectives is combined to support the enactment of policies that affect all components of the health care system. Hand surgeons' efforts to collaborate, advocate, adhere to standing guidelines, and conduct innovative research increase the effectiveness of policy and encourage improvement within the specialty.

INCIDENCE OF INJURY

The influence of health policy takes effect before patients reach the clinical setting. Hand injuries are the most common reason for a trip to the emergency room, accounting for more than 12% of all trauma cases in the United States.[12] Considering that traumatic injuries, and musculoskeletal disorders, such as carpal tunnel syndrome (CTS), often transpire in the workplace, the downstream effects of regulations to protect employee health are substantial.[13] For example, as part of the National Emphasis Program, representatives from the US Department of Labor's Occupational Health and Safety Administration (OSHA) periodically investigate high-risk workplaces for safety hazards that may lead to amputation injuries. Despite these efforts, Friedman and colleagues[14] reported that OSHA inspections rarely occurred within 60 days of an amputation event in the state of Illinois between 2000 and 2007 and that there were large discrepancies in amputation data between local and national databases. The authors recommended more stringent regulations for detection of workplace amputations. Incidentally, OSHA revised standing regulations in 2015 and now requires employers to report all work-related hospitalizations.[15] Continuous evaluation and reform of such policies can remove safety hazards, leading to improvements in public health.

Health care providers can contribute to upstream injury prevention efforts through collaboration with insurance companies and federal agencies, such as OSHA to confirm that accurate injury data are collected (**Fig. 2**). Better evidence improves understanding of the severity and economic impact of unintentional traumatic injuries. Additionally, hand surgeons may serve as detectives to identify any imminent threats to public health. A rise in gun violence, for example, presents unseen technical challenges to surgeons who treat the upper extremity.[16] Advances in gun-related research may shift policy efforts and funding to proportionally account for the impact of this emergent crisis on the health care system.[17]

Hand surgeons are a vital resource in the emergency setting. The demand for their services will increase in parallel with the rising occurrence of hand injuries. However, the evidence indicates that hand surgeons do not provide adequate care in trauma centers.[18–20] For example, a 2016 survey in New Jersey revealed that 64% of

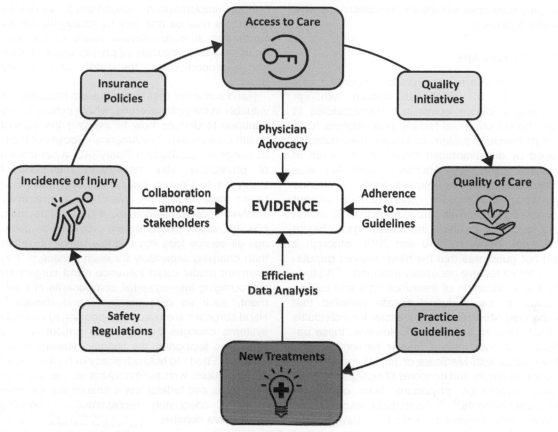

Fig. 1. Conceptual model.

hospitals had a hand specialist on call at all times for urgent consultations, whereas 84% offered elective hand surgery services. The authors discussed whether the high number of underinsured patients and lower reimbursements for emergency treatment contributed to this discrepancy.[21] Financial disincentives may discourage hand surgeons from working in the emergency room. The diminishing size of the surgical workforce is also a contributor to the shortage of on-call hand

surgeons.[19] Initiatives to reallocate resources on a statewide level and implement guidelines for the transfer of trauma patients to central hospitals may enable hand surgeons to expand their provision of care.[21] Additionally, validated triage systems already exist for burn and general trauma injuries. A similar system could be developed for better treatment of common hand injuries, such as amputations.[12] Implementation of policies to address the imbalance in allocation of hand

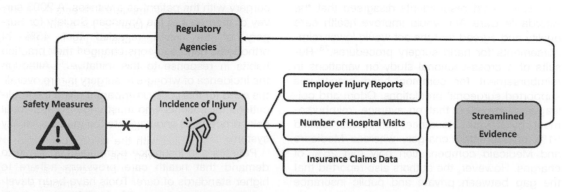

Fig. 2. Integration of evidence into safety regulation.

surgery resources will ensure that patients receive timely treatment.

ACCESS TO CARE

Unequal access to care has long been a major fault of the US health care system. Although growing evidence points out discrepancies in care based on social factors, policymakers have yet to devise a system to remove the obstacles faced by disadvantaged individuals in search of medical care. The Affordable Care Act was enacted in 2010 to expand health insurance coverage and improve quality of care without increasing costs. This helped more than 20 million previously uninsured individuals gain health coverage between 2010 and 2018, although it did not guarantee that the newly insured population would receive necessary treatment.[22] A study on the association of insurance type and patient access to carpal tunnel release revealed that expanded Medicaid made it easier for individuals to schedule an appointment. However, these patients still encountered greater barriers to care than those with Medicare or private insurance.[23] Lack of referrals and concerns of increased paperwork discourage physicians from caring for Medicaid patients.[24,25] Additionally, resource limitations may prevent patients from traveling the greater distance to a hand specialist who is willing to provide treatment.[26] Initiatives to simplify administrative tasks may increase opportunities for care. For example, widespread adoption of online health records and payment systems may streamline communication among patients, providers, and insurance companies.[27] The development of policy to oversee the transfer of care for nonurgent procedures will also help dismantle disparities responsible for preventing patients from receiving hand surgery.[26]

The financial effects of insurance reform extend from patients to providers. In a 2016 survey of members of the American Society for Surgery of the Hand, most respondents disagreed that the Affordable Care Act would improve health care quality and agreed that the act would lower reimbursements for hand surgery procedures.[28] Results of a cross-sectional study on variations in reimbursement for common hand procedures supported surgeons' predictions. Odom and colleagues[29] reported that on average, reimbursement by private insurance companies fulfilled 51% of submitted charges, whereas Medicare and Medicaid compensation only met 25% of charges. However, the authors also reported that the gap between private and public insurance reimbursement diminished overall during the study

period. Implementing value-based insurance structures may be one way to steady the recent fluctuations in reimbursement. Health care expenditures are better allocated if physician compensation is proportional to the quality of care they provide.

Hand surgeons' research on health disparities is valuable in the political arena, where policymakers continue to discuss how to improve the current health care system. The American Society of Plastic Surgeons established PlastyPAC, a committee of physicians who meet with members of Congress to discuss the clinical implications of health care legislation. Members are actively involved in conversations about bundled payment policies, which would require providers to package all service fees into a single payment, rather than charging separately for each service.[30] This payment model could influence hand surgery by discouraging less-essential components of treatment, such as postoperative hand therapy.[31] Hand surgeons are in a unique position to promote systems changes that increase patient access while also supporting the financial stability of the practice. Efforts to hold advocacy events and start conversations with policymakers at the community, state, and federal levels ensure that the specialty is adequately represented in ongoing health care debates.

QUALITY OF CARE

The evidence suggests that access to care alone does not guarantee high-quality treatment. At the turn of the twenty-first century, the National Academy of Medicine reported that more than 1 million injuries and 100,000 deaths occur because of medical mistakes each year.[32] This resulted in increased efforts to prevent malpractice across all areas of medicine, including hand surgery. In 1998, the American Academy of Orthopedic Surgeons announced the "Sign Your Site" campaign, requiring surgeons to sign their initials at the site of surgery with the patient as a witness. A 2003 survey of members of the American Society for Surgery of the Hand revealed that 45% of orthopedic hand surgeons changed their practice habits in response to this initiative.[33] Although the incidence of wrong-site surgery is rare overall, the need for this policy is apparent given the implications for patients who must undergo additional risky procedures and navigate the medical liability system.

Patients and insurance companies continue to demand that health care providers adhere to higher standards of care. Tools have been developed in several areas of medicine to assess aspects of health care structures and processes that affect patient outcomes.[34] Although quality metrics are often used to generate evidence of mortality or hospital readmissions, hand surgeons are more interested in how treatment decisions affect morbidity, especially after outpatient procedures. A collaborative quality initiative among nine hand surgery practices is currently underway. The goal of this endeavor is to elucidate how variations in processes across sites influence surgical outcomes. This information will be applied to set benchmarks for quality and establish evidence-based clinical guidelines.[35] A focus on quality also helps hand surgeons adapt to changes in health care structures. The Centers for Medicare & Medicaid Services established a value-based payment modifier program to penalize physicians who do not achieve a certain standard of care.[36] Surgeons should continue to generate evidence and update guidelines to maintain high quality of care while simultaneously reducing resource expenditures.[37]

Broader initiatives to improve health care quality also impact hand surgery. The Health Information Technology for Economic and Clinical Health Act of 2009 was implemented to incentivize adoption of a basic electronic health record (EHR). A nine-fold increase in its use at nonfederal acute hospitals was seen by 2015.[38] This portrays how policy can encourage widespread acceptance of quality initiatives and support consistent provision of care across hand surgery practices. The EHR can also be used to monitor physician adherence to guidelines and develop new methods for quality analysis.[39] Menendez and colleagues[40] used the EHR to identify "triggers," or predictors for adverse events after outpatient orthopedic surgery. For example, the administration of antibiotics within 3 months after surgery may indicate the development of surgical site infection. Considering that most adverse events after ambulatory surgery are not severe enough to warrant readmission, these data may elucidate whether a specific aspect of treatment causes postoperative complications. Additional research on automated, trigger-based methods could streamline efforts to monitor morbidity after hand surgery and provide evidence for novel outcomes analyses.

INNOVATION IN HAND SURGERY

Hand surgeons are skilled in a variety of techniques and tailor treatment plans to meet the unique needs of different patients. Nevertheless, contradicting evidence regarding the advantages of one procedure over another muddles the decision-making process for patients and providers alike. For example, the optimal treatment of CTS remains controversial. The American Academy of Orthopedic Surgeons published clinical practice guidelines recommending nonsurgical treatment for initial management of CTS, except in cases of denervation. Meanwhile, the literature suggests that earlier surgical intervention leads to better outcomes for patients with mild symptoms.[41] Even after a patient decides to undergo surgery, surgeons continue to debate whether open or endoscopic carpal tunnel release yields better results.[42] More research is warranted to determine the optimal CTS treatment based on the severity of the condition, patient needs, and surgeon skill.

Surgeons may be hesitant to adopt new technologies without evidence of the advantages over traditional methods, even when proven safe. For example, Yao[43] weighed the pros and cons of using a new technique for the treatment of a common hand problem, thumb carpometacarpal arthritis. Yao used the Mini-Tightrope suture button procedure for 4 years and observed good functional and patient-reported outcomes. Studies indicated that this procedure may lead to faster recovery and return to full activity than the common treatment, trapeziectomy. The authors also acknowledged the risks of the procedure, including index metacarpal fracture. However, they discussed how a second-generation technique greatly reduced the risks.[44] It is necessary for new procedures to be validated and refined on a smaller scale before adoption across the specialty. Additionally, evidence from long-term outcomes studies should be generated before the universal acceptance of novel surgical methods. At the same time, greater awareness of the inventive pursuits of hand surgeons may encourage innovation across the specialty and accelerate the integration of new techniques into practice.

New procedures often come with a steep learning curve and there is disagreement over who is responsible for their safe integration into practice. The consequences of inadequate training for new devices were exhibited during a 2017 Washington State Supreme Court case against the makers of the da Vinci Robotic Surgical System. A urologist's improper use of the device allegedly resulted in a patient's death. In response, the court declared that device manufacturers are legally obligated to ensure the safe adoption of their products. This measure is complementary to existing policies that require hospitals to confirm physicians' credentials and authorize their involvement in specific procedures.[45] Modern technology is a major contributor to innovation in hand surgery and similar decisions directly affect a surgeon's ability to explore novel techniques. Nevertheless, the adverse effects of inadequate evidence and lack of training must be addressed to avoid making hasty guidelines changes that put patient safety at risk. Progress often consists of two steps forward followed by one step back. It is worth considering how evidence can be generated more efficiently to confirm the safety of new procedures earlier in development. With the considerations of all stakeholders taken into account, progress in hand surgery will be steered toward a more linear trajectory.

SUMMARY

Hand surgeons view the intersection of health policy, clinical research, and patient experience from a rare perspective. Safety hazards and regulations upstream of the clinical setting contribute to the varied causes of hand conditions. Insurance reform influences patient access to care and a surgeon's capacity to provide treatment. Additionally, traditional methods for clinical research may or may not yield results that carry weight in the policy-making process. Surgeons' efforts to collaborate with policymakers within and beyond the health care setting encourage recognition of their patients' needs. Although investigators in hand surgery generate a wealth of impactful research each year, they should proceed with a heightened awareness of the implications of their findings on health policy.

DISCLOSURE

Dr. Kevin C. Chung receives funding from the National Institutes of Health and book royalties from Wolters Kluwer and Elsevier. He has received financial support from Axogen. The funding organizations had no role in the design and conduct of the study, including collection, management, analysis, and interpretation of the data.

REFERENCES

1. Research America. U.S. Investments in medical and health research and development 2013-2016. Arlington (VA): Research America; 2017. Available at: https://www.researchamerica.org/sites/default/files/Policy_Advocacy/2013-2017InvestmentReportFall2018.pdf.

2. Frieden TR. Evidence for health decision making: beyond randomized, controlled trials. N Engl J Med 2017;377(5):465–75.

3. Glasgow RE, Emmons KM. How can we increase translation of research into practice? Types of evidence needed. Annu Rev Public Health 2007;28:413–33.

4. Lenfant C. Shattuck lecture–clinical research to clinical practice–lost in translation? N Engl J Med 2003;349(9):868–74.

5. Brownson RC, Chriqui JF, Stamatakis KA. Understanding evidence-based public health policy. Am J Public Health 2009;99(9):1576–83.

6. Mendes E. The study that helped spur the U.S. stop-smoking movement. American Cancer Society; 2014. Available at: https://www.cancer.org/latest-news/the-study-that-helped-spur-the-us-stop-smoking-movement.html. Accessed June 15, 2019.

7. Paoletti L, Jardin B, Carpenter MJ, et al. Current status of tobacco policy and control. J Thorac Imaging 2012;27(4):213–9.

8. Clinical Practice Guideline Treating Tobacco Use and Dependence 2008 Update Panel, Liaisons, and Staff. A clinical practice guideline for treating tobacco use and dependence: 2008 update. A U.S. Public Health Service report. Am J Prev Med 2008;35(2):158–76.

9. Wei DH, Strauch RJ. Smoking and hand surgery. J Hand Surg Am 2013;38(1):176–9.

10. Stanek JJ, Renslow MA, Kalliainen LK. The effect of an educational program on opioid prescription patterns in hand surgery: a quality improvement program. J Hand Surg Am 2015;40(2):341–6.

11. Johnson SP, Chung KC, Zhong L, et al. Risk of prolonged opioid use among opioid-naive patients following common hand surgery procedures. J Hand Surg Am 2016;41(10):947–57.e3.

12. Maroukis BL, Chung KC, MacEachern M, et al. Hand trauma care in the United States: a literature review. Plast Reconstr Surg 2016;137(1):100e–11e.

13. Zwerling C, Daltroy LH, Fine LJ, et al. Design and conduct of occupational injury intervention studies: a review of evaluation strategies. Am J Ind Med 1997;32(2):164–79.

14. Friedman L, Krupczak C, Brandt-Rauf S, et al. Occupational amputations in Illinois 2000-2007: BLS vs. data linkage of trauma registry, hospital discharge, workers compensation databases and OSHA citations. Injury 2013;44(5):667–73.

15. OSHA announces new requirements for reporting severe injuries and updates list of industries exempt from record-keeping requirements 2014. US Department of Labor Web Site. Available at: https://www.osha.gov/news/newsreleases/national/09112014. Accessed June 10, 2020.

16. Omid R, Stone MA, Zalavras CG, et al. Gunshot wounds to the upper extremity. J Am Acad Orthop Surg 2019;27(7):e301–10.

17. Peetz AB, Haider A. Gun violence research and the profession of trauma surgery. AMA J Ethics 2018;20(5):475–82.

18. Rudkin SE, Oman J, Langdorf MI, et al. The state of ED on-call coverage in California. Am J Emerg Med 2004;22(7):575–81.

19. Rao MB, Lerro C, Gross CP. The shortage of on-call surgical specialist coverage: a national survey of emergency department directors. Acad Emerg Med 2010;17(12):1374–82.

20. Colen DL, Fox JP, Chang B, et al. Burden of hand maladies in US emergency departments. Hand (N Y). 2018;13(2):228–36.

21. Chung SY, Sood A, Granick MS. Disproportionate availability between emergency and elective hand coverage: a national trend? Eplasty 2016;16:e28.

22. Cohen RA, Martinez ME, Zammitti EP. Health insurance coverage: early release of estimates from the National Health Interview Survey, January-March 2018. National Center for Health Statistics; 2018. Available at: https://www.cdc.gov/nchs/nhis/releases.htm. Accessed June 17, 2019.

23. Kim CY, Wiznia DH, Wang YX, et al. The effect of insurance type on patient access to carpal tunnel release under the affordable care act. J Hand Surg Am 2016;41(4):503–9.

24. Berman S, Dolins J, Tang SF, et al. Factors that influence the willingness of private primary care pediatricians to accept more Medicaid patients. Pediatrics 2002;110(2 Pt 1):239–48.

25. Nguyen J, Anandasivam NS, Cooperman D, et al. Does Medicaid insurance provide sufficient access to pediatric orthopedic care under the affordable care act? Glob Pediatr Health 2019;6. 2333794X19831299.

26. Calfee RP, Shah CM, Canham CD, et al. The influence of insurance status on access to and utilization of a tertiary hand surgery referral center. J Bone Joint Surg Am 2012;94(23):2177–84.

27. Cutler D, Wikler E, Basch P. Reducing administrative costs and improving the health care system. N Engl J Med 2012;367(20):1875–8.

28. Shubinets V, Gerety PA, Pannucci CJ, et al. Attitude of hand surgeons toward Affordable Care Act: a survey of members of American Society for Surgery of the Hand. J Orthop 2017;14(1):38–44.

29. Odom EB, Hill E, Moore AM, et al. Lending a hand to health care disparities: a cross-sectional study of variations in reimbursement for common hand procedures. Hand (N Y) 2019. 1558944718825320.

30. Congress: bundled billing won't solve surprise billing. American Society of Plastic Surgeons; 2019. Available at: https://www.plasticsurgery.org/for-medical-professionals/advocacy/advocacy-news/congress-bundled-billing-wont-solve-surprise-billing. Accessed June 20, 2019.

31. Kamal RN, Hand Surgery Quality Consortium. Quality and value in an evolving health care landscape. J Hand Surg Am 2016;41(7):794–9.

32. Kohn LT, Corrigan J, Donaldson MS. To err is human: building a safer health system. Washington, DC: National Academies Press; 2000. p. 26–43.

33. Meinberg EG, Stern PJ. Incidence of wrong-site surgery among hand surgeons. J Bone Joint Surg Am 2003;85(2):193–7.

34. Chung KC, Shauver MJ. Measuring quality in health care and its implications for pay-for-performance initiatives. Hand Clin 2009;25(1):71–81, vii.

35. Billig JI, Kotsis SV, Chung KC. The next frontier of outcomes research: collaborative quality initiatives. Plast Reconstr Surg, in Press.

36. Centers for Medicare & Medicaid Services. Value-based payment modifier. 2015. Available at: https://www.cms.gov/Medicare/Medicare-Fee-for-Service-Payment/PhysicianFeedbackProgram/ValueBasedPaymentModifier.html. Accessed June 12, 2020.

37. Kamal RN, Kakar S, Ruch D, et al. Quality measurement: a primer for hand surgeons. J Hand Surg Am 2016;41(5):645–51.

38. Henry J, Plypchuk Y, Searcy S, et al. Adoption of electronic health record systems among U.S. Non-federal acute care hospitals: 2008-2015. Washington, DC: ONC Data Brief, no.35. Office of the National Coordinator for Health Information Technology; 2016. Available at: https://dashboard.healthit.gov/evaluations/data-briefs/non-federal-acute-care-hospital-ehr-adoption-2008-2015.php.

39. Jha AK. Meaningful use of electronic health records: the road ahead. JAMA 2010;304(15):1709–10.

40. Menendez ME, Janssen SJ, Ring D. Electronic health record-based triggers to detect adverse events after outpatient orthopaedic surgery. BMJ Qual Saf 2016;25(1):25–30.

41. Ono S, Clapham PJ, Chung KC. Optimal management of carpal tunnel syndrome. Int J Gen Med 2010;3:255–61.

42. Wagner ER, Chung KC. Commentary on "our surgical experience: open versus endoscopic carpal tunnel surgery. J Hand Surg Am 2018;43(9):862–3.

43. Yao J. Suture-button suspensionplasty for the treatment of thumb carpometacarpal joint arthritis. Hand Clin 2012;28(4):579–85.

44. Yao J, Lashgari D. Thumb basal joint: utilizing new technology for the treatment of a common problem. J Hand Ther 2014;27(2):127–32 [quiz: 133].

45. Pradarelli JC, Thornton JP, Dimick JB. Who is responsible for the safe introduction of new surgical technology?: an important legal precedent from the Da Vinci surgical system trials. JAMA Surg 2017;152(8):717–8.

Bringing Evidence into Practice in Hand Surgery

Jennifer F. Waljee, MD, MPH*, Kevin C. Chung, MD, MS

KEYWORDS

• Implementation • Dissemination • Hand surgery

KEY POINTS

• The diffusion of evidence into practice and policy is complex and is influenced by social, environmental, cultural, and behavioral factors.
• The rigor of the available evidence to guide practice in hand surgery often is variable.
• Lessons learned from implementation and dissemination science and the emergence of learning health systems will improve the application of evidence toward clinical care and policy to enhance the delivery of care of the hand and upper extremity.

INTRODUCTION

To achieve high-value care, it is critical that health care systems adopt and implement the best scientific evidence, capture relevant outcomes to benchmark progress, and leverage their informational infrastructure to enhance clinical performance. Health care in the United States, however, is marked by accelerating costs, an expanding and aging population, and competing economic demands. In addition, health care outcomes continue to lag behind other developed health care systems.[1,2] Quality and accessibility of health care in the United States are variable, and the best available evidence often does not reach key stakeholders and end users, including clinicians, policy makers, and ultimately patients.[3] This review examines critical factors that influence the translation of evidence into clinical practice and policy: evaluation of current evidence, disseminating best practices, identifying organizational readiness and barriers to change, and creating sustainable systems for quality improvement.

EVALUATING THE EVIDENCE

Evidence-based practice describes the application of clinical science toward patient care,

accounting for clinical expertise, patient values, and the contextual aspects of the health care system.[4–6] Evidence-based practice also provides a framework for clinicians, researchers, and policy makers to consider the value of the available evidence, including its limitations, applications, and gaps. These evaluation frameworks are critical to identify those health care interventions that are expected to bring the greatest value if adopted as well as those that bring less value and should be avoided.[7,8] Numerous organizations have developed standardized approaches to assessing the evidence base, such as the National Academy of Medicine (NAM), the US Preventive Services Task Force, and the Grading of Recommendations Assessment, Development and Evaluation (GRADE) working group. For example, the NAM published *Clinical Practice Guidelines We Can Trust* in 2011,[7] detailing criteria by which available evidence could be considered to develop clinical guidelines, such as transparency and disclosure of conflicts of interest. The GRADE working group also has developed a standardized approach to assess the quality of available evidence by integrating criteria, including bias, precision, consistency, and outcome selection.[9,10] Finally, evidence may also be evaluated using the Cochrane Effective Practice and Organisation of

Section of Plastic Surgery, Department of Surgery, Michigan Medicine, 1500 East Medical Center Drive, 2130 Taubman Center, SPC 5340, Ann Arbor, MI 48109-5340, USA
* Corresponding author.
E-mail address: filip@med.umich.edu

Hand Clin 36 (2020) 131–136
https://doi.org/10.1016/j.hcl.2020.01.014

Care (EPOC) criteria for levels of evidence for health systems interventions. These guidelines provide a framework for identifying relevant information that can be gleaned from scientific studies, creating transparency around potential sources of bias and opportunities for generalizability of the findings. The Cochrane EPOC criteria also have been tailored toward a variety of study designs testing health care interventions, including randomized controlled trials, interrupted time series analyses, and controlled predesisgns/postdesigns.

Specific to hand surgery, the rigor of the available evidence varies widely. For example, a recent study demonstrates that the studies of high-level evidence, such as randomized controlled trials and prospective comparative studies, account for only 11% of published articles.[11] Although the percentage is increasing, a vast majority of articles published in hand surgery fall into categories of lower evidence, including case series and single-center, retrospective assessments without comparison groups.[12] Finally, the evidence base often hovers around a few common conditions. For example, a recent study noted that approximately 30% of all publications in hand surgery were focused on distal radius fractures, flexor tendon injuries, and carpal tunnel syndrome.[13] As a discipline, hand surgery is unique in the broad range of acute and chronic conditions encompassing a range of anatomic areas. As such, it may be challenging to amass an adequate number of patients with any given condition with sufficient homogeneity for a comparative study with sufficient power to identify differences in treatment groups. In addition, it is likely that more rigorous designs that include randomization, placebo groups, or blinding are challenging to conduct in surgical care due to ethical and logistical reasons. Nonetheless, a transparent and candid evaluation of the available evidence is necessary to identify those aspects of clinical practice that yield the greatest benefit for patients.

DISSEMINATION AND IMPLEMENTATION

Despite immense effort and funding directed toward discovery and innovation in health care, it typically is decades from the time of development to implementation, and few interventions ultimately are incorporated into care.[14,15] To understand and overcome these gaps, the disciplines of dissemination and implementation science describe the investigation into translation of knowledge into clinical practice.[16] Implementation science specifically refers to the study of the processes by which evidence-based interventions are integrated into routine clinical care, whereas dissemination science describes the examination of the processes of bringing evidence to the attention of key stakeholders, health care systems, and end users.[17] Dissemination describes the process in which evidence is presented to key stakeholders and a target audience. In medicine, dissemination strategies traditionally have relied on passive dissemination models, including publications in peer-reviewed journals and presentations at scientific meetings.[18] Although this approach is common, it places the burden of practice change on the practitioner and often is insufficient.[19] In contrast, active strategies to disseminate evidence couple education with intentional aspects of education, such as academic detailing models and coaching.[20] The goals of implementation and dissemination science are to improve the uptake of evidence-based strategies by identifying and addressing barriers within an organization or health care setting. In addition, implementation and dissemination science aims to understand the ways in which interventions are appropriately, or inappropriately, adopted into practice in order to promote high-value health care. Finally, implementation and dissemination science seek to identify pathways for sustainable change in clinical care.

The critical components of evaluating the effectiveness of the dissemination and implementation of best practices in health care systems include

1. Defining the critical gaps in care or quality
2. Defining the care intervention to be implemented
3. Identifying a conceptual framework to inform the approach for testing and measuring outcomes
4. Presenting the key stakeholders and understanding the organization's readiness for change
5. Establishing the strategy to implement/deimplement care
6. Measuring and evaluating outcomes[21]

Defining the critical gaps in care and identifying potential interventions to overcome these gaps are achieved through a systematic review of the available evidence and evaluating the evidence using established frameworks, as described previously. This approach ensures the importance of the evaluation and the potential for public health impact as well as the readiness of the intervention for clinical care.

Conceptual Frameworks

Given the complexity of relationships and organizations in health care, conceptual frameworks are essential to organize the potential influencing factors and underlying mechanisms that relate to the implementation of interventions into clinical practice in a meaningful way.[16,21] These frameworks guide the evaluation of the implementation of the intervention and inform hypotheses for testing regarding the barriers and facilitators of implementation. Conceptual frameworks may center on individuals, or evaluate factors at the level of the organization.

Numerous conceptual frameworks have been described to encompass that factors and relationships that underlie evidence dissemination and implementation. For example, the diffusion of innovations theory describes the mechanisms by which innovation is adopted through 5 attributes: relative advantage, compatibility, complexity, trialability, and observability.[22] In this model, interventions that have clear advantage are simple, align with established values, may be tested in a limited trial, and have observable results. As a result, these interventions are more likely to be adopted than those that do not have these favorable attributes.[23] The theoretical domains framework describes a systematic approach across multiple domains to understand the mechanisms that underlie interventions aimed at behavior change.[24] Domains include

1. Knowledge of risks, alternatives, and advantages
2. Training and experience
3. Social/professional role and identity
4. Beliefs about capabilities
5. Beliefs about consequences
6. Motivation and goals
7. Memory, attention, and decision processes
8. Environmental context and resources
9. Social influences
10. Emotion
11. Behavioral regulation
12. Nature of the behaviors[24]

This framework has been used previously to describe provider behaviors and response to interventions designed to promote change in clinical care across a variety of other conditions, such as the management of cardiopulmonary disease, reporting of medical errors, and adherence to evidence based guidelines.[25–28] The Consolidated Framework for Implementation Research (CFIR) spans multiple theories across 5 interrelated domains that influence the implementation of an intervention:

- Intervention characteristics (evidence base, advantage, adaptability, trialability, and complexity)

- The environmental setting (patient needs and resources, organizational network, social influence, and external policy)
- The organizational setting (structural attributes, communication, culture, climate, and readiness)
- Stakeholder attributes (knowledge, self-efficacy, stage of change, and engagement)
- Implementation strategy (planning, engaging, executing, reflecting, and evaluating)[29,30]

The CFIR provides an expansive approach to evaluating the process of implementation across any phase and provides a common foundation for comparing findings across studies.

Identifying Key Stakeholders and Organizational Readiness

Identifying key stakeholders and end users is critical to understand the process by which evidence is implemented into practice. Stakeholders and end users may include not only clinicians and patients but also policy makers, administrators, funders, payers, and researchers and may have variable preferences, experiences, knowledge, and perceptions of gaps in care and potential interventions.[31] Each of these factors may influence the readiness for change in clinical care. Similarly, the attributes and readiness of an organization influence the propensity for implementation of interventions and may not be the sum of the readiness of individuals within an organization.[32] Instead, organizations reflect coordinated behavioral change and may be dependent on the workforce quantity and complement, communication, and policies and incentives.

Defining Implementation Strategies and Capturing Outcomes

Appropriate targets for strategies focused on implementation include those that are demonstrated to be most effective compared with other options in high-quality evidence or those that are shown to be more efficient without compromising outcomes. Conversely, practices that are not effective, not efficient, or are no longer necessary could be considered to deimplement.[33] Strategies for implementation can be considered using standardized tools to capture sufficient detail and consistency across studies.[34,35] For example, the Template for Intervention Description and Replication guide was developed in 2014 to enhance the reporting of intervention studies for transparency and replicability of research findings.[36] Alternatively, the Standards for Reporting Implementation Studies Statement guidelines provide a rationale and standards for reporting intervention implementation studies.[37]

Critical outcomes include the acceptability of interventions to key stakeholders (eg, clinicians and patients), the feasibility of executing the intervention in routine clinical care, the fidelity of the intervention, and the appropriateness of the intervention.[38] Appropriateness describes the relevance of the intervention to the practice setting or to end users and key stakeholders.[39] In contrast, fidelity describes the extent to which an intervention is applied in clinical care in its intended way. In addition, it also is important to assess variation in the adoption of the intervention across the organization by groups or region, alongside the cost of the intervention, to identify areas in which this is high and those in which adoption has lagged by group or region. Finally, examining the sustainability of intervention uptake over time is critical to understand opportunities for enhancing care going forward.

EFFECTIVE MODELS FOR CLINICAL CHANGE: LEARNING HEALTH SYSTEMS

It is critical to understand the attributes of organizations that can integrate best practices, evaluate effectiveness, and refine care efficiently. Learning health systems are defined as health care delivery systems that integrate research, data science, and continuous quality improvement in order to gain knowledge and enhance patient outcomes.[40] The hallmark of learning health care systems is the integration of health care and research simultaneously to leverage shared experiences and perspectives.[41] Distinct from traditional research models, which occur linearly, learning health systems evaluate opportunities for care improvement cyclically. In this way, knowledge is obtained through research and immediately applied toward clinical care to enhance outcomes (**Fig. 1**).[42,43]

A common example of learning health systems in practice includes collaborative quality-improvement (CQI) programs. CQI programs are funded by large payers and provide incentives for providers to participate in quality assessment and improvement. In addition, CQI programs facilitate collaboration across health care systems through a shared infrastructure and typically are organized around a specific medical or surgical condition.[44,45] Although each program is tailored to the nuances of clinical care, CQI programs all share 4 critical elements: rigorous data, timely feedback, transparent reporting, and collaborative improvement. Within the programs, each hospital collects clinical data regarding outcomes of interest or relevant processes of care. Data are

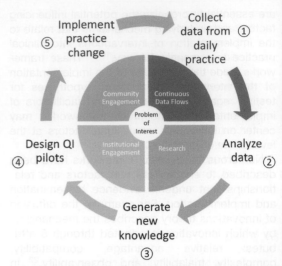

Fig. 1. Processes of a learning health system. QI, quality improvement. (*From* Howard R, Vu J, Lee J, et al. A Pathway for Developing Postoperative Opioid Prescribing Best Practices. Ann Surg 2020;271(1):86–93; with permission.)

maintained in clinical registries that account for case mix and patient factors. For example, the Michigan Society of Thoracic and Cardiovascular Surgeons leverages a data collection registry developed by the Society of Thoracic Surgeons to capture clinical events, such as postoperative complications and mortality. Providers regularly review individualized and aggregate performance data and identify opportunities for quality-improvement strategies. For example, an analysis of processes of care within the Michigan Bariatric Surgery Collaborative revealed variation in the use of inferior vena cava (IVC) filters to prevent postoperative pulmonary embolism. The IVC filters had no clear efficacy and were associated with significant risks.[46] Through the learning health system structure of the collaborative to evaluate and disseminate this evidence, the use of IVC filters and their associated complications declined precipitously.[47] The effectiveness of CQI programs in translating evidence into practice in real time indicates that these types of learning health system models with likely will be the standard going forward to promote high-value care.

SUMMARY

Effective integration of best practices and high-level evidence is critical to optimize the quality of care in the United States and reduce costs. Diffusion and uptake of innovation in clinical practice are complex, however, and demand close study to identify the strategies that yield the greatest effect in improving the implementation of high-value interventions and the deimplementation of less valuable care. Dissemination and implementation science aims to improve health outcomes through identifying effective strategies for implementing best evidence and define the barriers and facilitators to implementation success.[48] The real-world consequences of successful dissemination and implementation include the emergence of learning health systems, which can harness these properties and principles for continuous improvement. Going forward, these efforts will enhance the efficiency of translating research into practice, improve the care of patients, and promote wellness and public health.

DISCLOSURE

The authors have nothing to disclose.

REFERENCES

1. Shrank WH, Rogstad TL, Parekh N. Waste in the US health care system: estimated costs and potential for savings. JAMA 2019. [Epub ahead of print].

2. Dieleman JL, Baral R, Birger M, et al. US spending on personal health care and public health, 1996-2013. JAMA 2016;316(24):2627–46.

3. America CoQHCi, Medicine IO. Crossing the quality Chasm: a new health system for the 21st century. Washington, DC: National Academies Press; 2001.

4. Guyatt GH, Rennie D, Meade MO, et al. Users' guide to the medical literature: a manual for evidence-based practice. 2nd edition. New York: McGraw-Hill Education; 2008.

5. Sackett DL, Strauss SE, Richardson WS, et al. Evidence-based medicine: how to practice and teach EBM. Edinburgh (Scotland): Churchill Livingston; 2000.

6. Sackett DL, Rosenberg WM, Gray JA, et al. Evidence based medicine: what it is and what it isn't. BMJ 1996;312(7023):71–2.

7. Medicine IO. Clinical practice guidelines we can trust. Washington, DC: National Academies Press; 2011.

8. Medicine IO. Value in health care. Accounting for cost, quality, safety, and innovation: workshop summary. Washington, DC: National Academies Press; 2010.

9. Zhang Y, Alonso-Coello P, Guyatt GH, et al. GRADE guidelines: 19. Assessing the certainty of evidence in the importance of outcomes or values and preferences-Risk of bias and indirectness. J Clin Epidemiol 2019;111:94–104.

10. Zhang Y, Coello PA, Guyatt GH, et al. GRADE guidelines: 20. Assessing the certainty of evidence in the importance of outcomes or values and preferences-inconsistency, imprecision, and other domains. J Clin Epidemiol 2019;111:83–93.

11. Sugrue CM, Joyce CW, Sugrue RM, et al. Trends in the level of evidence in clinical hand surgery research. Hand (N Y) 2016;11(2):211–5.

12. Rosales RS, Reboso-Morales L, Martin-Hidalgo Y, et al. Level of evidence in hand surgery. BMC Res Notes 2012;5:665.

13. Lemme NJ, Johnston BR, Smith BC, et al. Common topics of publication and levels of evidence in the current hand surgery literature. J Hand Microsurg 2019;11(1):14–7.

14. Balas EA, Chapman WW. Road map for diffusion of innovation in health care. Health Aff 2018;37(2):198–204.

15. Kirchner JE, Smith JL, Powell BJ, et al. Getting a clinical innovation into practice: an introduction to implementation strategies. Psychiatry Res 2019;283:112467.

16. Proctor EK, Landsverk J, Aarons G, et al. Implementation research in mental health services: an emerging science with conceptual, methodological, and training challenges. Adm Policy Ment Health 2009;36(1):24–34.

17. Holtrop JS, Rabin BA, Glasgow RE. Dissemination and implementation science in primary care research and practice: contributions and opportunities. J Am Board Fam Med 2018;31(3):466–78.

18. Munn Z, Stern C, Porritt K, et al. Evidence transfer: ensuring end users are aware of, have access to, and understand the evidence. Int J Evid Based Healthc 2018;16(2):83–9.

19. Estabrooks PA, Brownson RC, Pronk NP. Dissemination and implementation science for public health professionals: an overview and call to action. Prev Chronic Dis 2018;15:E162.

20. Wensing M, Grol R. Knowledge translation in health: how implementation science could contribute more. BMC Med 2019;17(1):88.

21. Proctor EK, Powell BJ, Baumann AA, et al. Writing implementation research grant proposals: ten key ingredients. Implement Sci 2012;7:96.

22. Dearing JW, Cox JG. Diffusion of innovations theory, principles, and practice. Health Aff 2018;37(2):183–90.

23. Scott SD, Plotnikoff RC, Karunamuni N, et al. Factors influencing the adoption of an innovation: an examination of the uptake of the Canadian Heart Health Kit (HHK). Implement Sci 2008;3:41.

24. Francis JJ, O'Connor D, Curran J. Theories of behaviour change synthesised into a set of theoretical groupings: introducing a thematic series on the theoretical domains framework. Implement Sci 2012;7:35.

25. Lawton R, Heyhoe J, Louch G, et al. Using the Theoretical Domains Framework (TDF) to understand adherence to multiple evidence-based indicators in primary care: a qualitative study. Implement Sci 2016;11:113.

26. Skoien W, Page K, Parsonage W, et al. Use of the Theoretical Domains Framework to evaluate factors driving successful implementation of the Accelerated Chest pain Risk Evaluation (ACRE) project. Implement Sci 2016;11(1):136.

27. Alqubaisi M, Tonna A, Strath A, et al. Quantifying behavioural determinants relating to health professional reporting of medication errors: a cross-sectional survey using the Theoretical Domains Framework. Eur J Clin Pharmacol 2016;72(11): 1401–11.

28. Kisala PA, Tulsky DS. Opportunities for CAT applications in medical rehabilitation: development of targeted item banks. J Appl Meas 2010;11(3):315–30.

29. Keith RE, Crosson JC, O'Malley AS, et al. Using the Consolidated Framework for Implementation Research (CFIR) to produce actionable findings: a rapid-cycle evaluation approach to improving implementation. Implement Sci 2017;12(1):15.

30. Kirk MA, Kelley C, Yankey N, et al. A systematic review of the use of the Consolidated Framework for Implementation Research. Implement Sci 2016; 11:72.

31. Mendel P, Meredith LS, Schoenbaum M, et al. Interventions in organizational and community context: a framework for building evidence on dissemination and implementation in health services research. Adm Policy Ment Health 2008;35(1–2):21–37.

32. Weiner BJ, Amick H, Lee SY. Conceptualization and measurement of organizational readiness for change: a review of the literature in health services research and other fields. Med Care Res Rev 2008;65(4):379–436.

33. McKay VR, Morshed AB, Brownson RC, et al. Letting go: conceptualizing intervention de-implementation in public health and social service settings. Am J Community Psychol 2018;62(1–2):189–202.

34. Improved Clinical Effectiveness through Behavioural Research Group. Designing theoretically-informed implementation interventions. Implement Sci 2006;1:4.

35. Bhattacharyya O, Reeves S, Garfinkel S, et al. Designing theoretically-informed implementation interventions: fine in theory, but evidence of effectiveness in practice is needed. Implement Sci 2006;1:5.

36. Hoffmann TC, Glasziou PP, Boutron I, et al. Better reporting of interventions: template for intervention description and replication (TIDieR) checklist and guide. BMJ 2014;348:g1687.

37. Pinnock H, Barwick M, Carpenter CR, et al. Standards for Reporting Implementation Studies (StaRI) statement. BMJ 2017;356:i6795.

38. Proctor E, Silmere H, Raghavan R, et al. Outcomes for implementation research: conceptual distinctions, measurement challenges, and research agenda. Adm Policy Ment Health 2011;38(2):65–76.

39. Weiner BJ, Lewis CC, Stanick C, et al. Psychometric assessment of three newly developed implementation outcome measures. Implement Sci 2017;12(1):108.

40. Medicine IO. The learning health system and its innovation collaboratives. Washington, DC: 2011.

41. Deans KJ, Sabihi S, Forrest CB. Learning health systems. Semin Pediatr Surg 2018;27(6):375–8.

42. Krumholz HM. Big data and new knowledge in medicine: the thinking, training, and tools needed for a learning health system. Health Aff 2014;33(7): 1163–70.

43. Medicine IO. Best care at lower cost: the path to continuously learning health care in America. Washington, DC: 2013.

44. Birkmeyer NJ, Share D, Campbell DA Jr, et al. Partnering with payers to improve surgical quality: the Michigan plan. Surgery 2005;138(5):815–20.

45. Birkmeyer NJ, Birkmeyer JD. Strategies for improving surgical quality–should payers reward excellence or effort? N Engl J Med 2006;354(8): 864–70.

46. Birkmeyer NJ, Finks JF, English WJ, et al. Risks and benefits of prophylactic inferior vena cava filters in patients undergoing bariatric surgery. J Hosp Med 2013;8(4):173–7.

47. Share DA, Campbell DA, Birkmeyer N, et al. How a regional collaborative of hospitals and physicians in Michigan cut costs and improved the quality of care. Health Aff (Millwood) 2011;30(4):636–45.

48. Grimshaw J, Eccles M, Thomas R, et al. Toward evidence-based quality improvement. Evidence (and its limitations) of the effectiveness of guideline dissemination and implementation strategies 1966-1998. J Gen Intern Med 2006;21(Suppl 2):S14–20.

Using Evidence for Hand Surgery
How to Practice Evidence-Based Hand Surgery Care

Kristine A. Huynh, BS[a,1], Kevin C. Chung, MD, MS[b,*]

KEYWORDS

- Evidence-based medicine • Evidence-based practice • Level of evidence • Research
- Critical appraisal

KEY POINTS

- Evidence-based practice (EBP) requires the integration of 3 components: the highest level of evidence available, the physician's cumulative experience and expertise, and patient preferences and values.
- The shift towards EBP aims to decrease variability in practice and optimize patient care through creating evidence-based, standardized guidelines.
- Evidence must be assessed for bias regardless of its placement in the hierarchy of evidence because every study is subjected to some form of bias.

INTRODUCTION

Evidence-based practice (EBP) is the practice of evidence-based medicine (EBM), a new paradigm in medicine that stemmed from concerns regarding quality of care and inefficiency of the healthcare system of the United States.[1–3] EBM, introduced in 1991, is defined as "the conscientious, explicit, and judicious use of current best evidence in making decisions about the care of the individual patient."[4,5] EBP is the integration of the best evidence gathered from a systematic search with the physician's accumulated experience, as well as patient preferences and values.[4,6,7] EBP has helped providers create standardized, evidence-based protocols and use real-time data to make clinical decisions.[2] Moreover, EBP tackles the problem of broad variations in care stemming from "underuse, overuse, and misuse" of diagnostic and therapeutic services.[8] EBP increases both transparency and accountability, enhancing overall quality of care.[9,10] For example, the EBP method has been used to update guidelines in preoperative and postoperative management of sternal wounds after open heart surgery to decrease the incidence of sternal wound infections.[11] EBP yielded changes in preoperative skin preparation, antibiotic prophylaxis, blood glucose control, wound care management, and hand hygiene. After the implementation of new institution-specific guidelines, there was a reduction in sternal wound infections, which substantially impacts patient morbidity, length of stay, and cost of care. In addition to revising protocols, EBP was also used to consolidate and decrease variability in acute and

[a] Oakland University William Beaumont School of Medicine, Rochester, MI, USA; [b] Section of Plastic Surgery, Department of Surgery, University of Michigan Medical School, Michigan Medicine Comprehensive Hand Center, University of Michigan, 2130 Taubman Center, SPC 5340, 1500 East Medical Center Drive, Ann Arbor, MI 48109-5340, USA
[1] Present address: NCRC, 2800 Plymouth Road, Building 14, G200, Ann Arbor, MI 48109.
* Corresponding author.
E-mail address: kecchung@umich.edu
Twitter: @kecchung (K.C.C.)

Hand Clin 36 (2020) 137–144
https://doi.org/10.1016/j.hcl.2019.12.001

chronic wound management among general surgeons, plastic surgeons, and hand surgeons.[12] This article discusses in detail the steps of the EBP process and applies them in a clinical scenario to better explain how to practice evidence-based hand surgery care.

CLINICAL SCENARIO

A 60-year-old, right-handed man was referred to the hand clinic by his family care physician for inability to extend his right finger. The patient noticed a few painless nodules on his right hand a few years ago. Recently, he has been experiencing stiffness that hinders his daily activities. Physical examination revealed nodules at the base of the ring and little digits on his right hand; the left hand remains unaffected. Dupuytren contracture (DC) was subsequently diagnosed, and treatment options were discussed. The patient expressed interest in minimally invasive treatments and preferred to return to work as early as possible.

DC is a slow progressive fibroproliferative disease of the palmar fascia.[13] The exact etiology of DC is unknown; genetics, ethnicity, sex, age, and certain environmental factors have been proposed as associated risks in development of the disease.[14] The initial presentation is often unnoticed, presenting as a painless thickened nodule. However, it insidiously progresses to joint stiffness and loss of extension at the metacarpal phalangeal joint, proximal interphalangeal joint, or both.

STEPS TO EVIDENCE-BASED PRACTICE

The 6 steps to practicing evidence-based medicine is outlined in **Fig. 1**. The authors discuss the clinical scenario proposed in the preceding paragraphs by walking through each step of the EBP process.

Assess the Patient

The first step of the EBP process is to evaluate the patient and determine the type of clinical question regarding the patient's care. These questions can be divided into 4 broad categories: therapy, prognosis, diagnosis, and economic/decision analysis. For example, if a provider is interested in comparing different treatment options, this is a therapy question. If the provider wants to understand the clinical outcomes after fasciectomy, this is a prognosis question. Diagnosis questions can investigate the sensitivity or specificity of a clinical tool, such as using dual x-ray absorptiometry scan to diagnose osteoporosis.[15] Economic/decision analysis questions relate the costs and benefits of different treatment options, such as determining a low-cost approach to the management of possible scaphoid fractures with optimal patient outcomes.

In our clinical scenario, we have a 60-year-old man with DC of his dominant hand, which significantly limits his daily activities. The patient prefers a minimally invasive intervention for these new lesions with an earlier return to work and daily activity. Invasive treatment options consist of limited fasciectomy, total fasciectomy, and dermofasciectomy, whereas minimally invasive treatments include percutaneous needle aponeurotomy or fasciotomy (PNF) and collagenase *Clostridium histolyticum* injections (CCH).[16,17] Our clinical topic regards therapy and determining which minimally invasive intervention is appropriate for this patient.

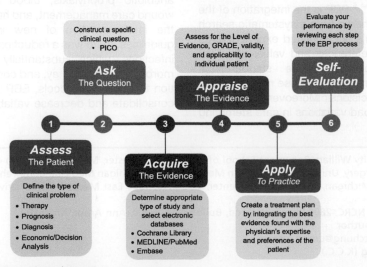

Fig. 1. Steps to evidence-based practice.

Ask the Question

The second step of the EBP process is to develop a specific clinical question. PICO is a framing tool available to physicians to build a clear, focused clinical question. PICO stands for Patient/Problem, Intervention, Comparison Intervention, and Outcomes. Increasing the specificity of each PICO component prevents providers from wasting time assessing irrelevant articles during the literature search. For example, a poor question for this clinical scenario is "What is the best therapy for Dupuytren contracture?" This question is too broad and will result in many unrelated findings. The proposed question also does not address the patient population or capture the patient's values or preferred type of treatment. Using the PICO framework, an appropriate clinical question for this case is "In middle-age men with Dupuytren contractures, does percutaneous needle fasciotomy compared with collagenase *C histolyticum* injections lead to faster functional improvement?" This question is clinically relevant, specific, and answerable.

Acquire the Evidence

In EBP, acquiring the evidence can be divided into 2 aspects: the type of evidence and the electronic databases. The appropriate type of evidence is determined by the type of clinical question. Therapy questions are best answered through randomized controlled trials (RCTs); however, RCTs are limited in surgery due to feasibility of randomization, such as ethical concerns, emergency settings, or palliative care.[9,18] For example, Slim[6] performed a search in the *Cochrane Database of Systematic Reviews* (CDSR) in 2003 and found that only 169 (5.3%) of 3151 total systematic reviews were surgical. When systematic reviews are unavailable, the best evidence comes from nonexperimental studies, such as nonrandomized case-control studies, cohort studies, or qualitative studies. When RCTs are unavailable, therapy questions can be answered with prospective cohort studies.[6,19] Prospective cohort studies are also appropriate when inquiring about the prognosis of a disease. Diagnostic studies to evaluate novel tools are best answered with cross-sectional or prospective cohort studies, whereas economic/decision analysis questions can be answered with cost-analysis studies.

Databases frequently used are the Cochrane Library, MEDLINE, and Embase. The Cochrane Collaborative maintains the Cochrane Library, which consists of many resources available to practice evidence-based care. The most notable resource within the library is the CDSR, which consists of high-quality reviews of any topic related to health care and medicine. Each review follows a strict, publicized protocol and undergoes a rigorous review process by the Cochrane Review Group before publication.[20,21] MEDLINE, created by the US National Library of Medicine, is a database of mainly life science articles with a special concentration in biomedicine. This database contains articles from more than 5200 journals worldwide in more than 40 different languages.[22] In 2018, more than 900,000 citations were added to MEDLINE. MEDLINE articles are the primary component of the PubMed archive. PubMed has several features to improve the specificity of the search process. For example, users can search for a specific citation or journal or use Clinical Queries to narrow the search by subject or clinical study category (eg, diagnosis, prognosis) or type (eg, systematic reviews).[23] Embase has biomedical articles dating back to 1947 and contains more than 32 million articles from more than 8500 journals.[24] Compared with MEDLINE, Embase contains more European journals and pharmaceutical papers. Although the same articles often overlap across these 3 commonly used databases, it is still important for users to use more than one database for a comprehensive search and gather all the best evidence available.

In our clinical scenario, we completed the search using the databases mentioned previously and found zero systematic reviews or meta-analyses of RCTs, a few RCTs comparing PNF and CCH, and many retrospective reviews investigating clinical outcomes following PNF or CCH for DC.

Appraise the Evidence

After acquiring the best evidence available, the next step is to assess the findings for level of evidence; Grading of Recommendations Assessment, Development, and Evaluation (GRADE); validity; and applicability to this individual patient. The hierarchy of evidence ranks studies based on the quality of evidence and risk of bias (**Fig. 2**). High-quality RCTs and systematic reviews or meta-analyses of RCTs are at the top of the pyramid, whereas case series and editorial or expert opinions are at the bottom. Systematic reviews or meta-analyses of RCTs are considered the highest quality of evidence because if done correctly, the pooled data provide the reader with an unbiased summary of the current evidence available. Studies completed in a nonsystematic manner, such as editorials and expert opinions, are more prone to bias, which places these articles at the bottom of the pyramid. In addition to the pyramid scale, studies can be classified by their level of

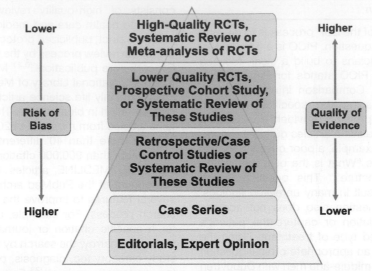

Fig. 2. Hierarchy of evidence.

evidence. The level of evidence, originally proposed by the Canadian Task Force on the Periodic Health Examination, is a classification system that correlates specific study design to levels I to V.[25] The level of evidence is often assigned by the authors or the publisher of a journal based on publicly available evidence rating scales. For example, the evidence rating scales of the American Society of Plastic Surgeons (ASPS) for therapeutic, diagnostic, and prognostic studies are in **Tables 1–3**. A study design can differ in level of evidence based on the clinical subject. For example, a prospective cohort study can be classified as Level I if it is regarding the prognosis of a disease or Level II if it is regarding therapeutic intervention. Although studies at the top of the hierarchy pyramid and higher levels of evidence have a low risk of bias, all studies are susceptible to some form of bias. All evidence must be stringently evaluated for potential biases, types of errors, the power of the study, and overall validity of study regardless of their level of evidence or place in the hierarchy of evidence. The GRADE associates strength of recommendation in clinical practice to a grade based on the quality of evidence. This system does not degrade lower levels of evidence, such as levels II to IV, if the results are consistent. For example, the grade practice recommendations of the ASPS are in **Table 4**.

Our search revealed that both PNF and CCH are safe and effective minimally invasive treatment options with low complication rates for patients with mild or moderate DC. RCTs demonstrated that CCH is not superior to PNF in terms of clinical outcomes at 1- or 2-year follow-up. Skov and

Table 1
The ASPS evidence rating scale for therapeutic studies

Level of Evidence	Qualifying Studies
I	High-quality, multicentered or single-centered, randomized controlled trial with adequate power; or systematic review of these studies
II	Lesser-quality, randomized controlled trial; prospective cohort or comparative study; or systematic review of these studies
III	Retrospective cohort or comparative study; case-control study; or systematic review of these studies
IV	Case series with pre/posttest; or only posttest
V	Expert opinion developed via consensus process; case report or clinical example; or evidence based on physiology, bench research or "first principles"

From the American Society of Plastic Surgeons. Available at: https://www.plasticsurgery.org/documents/medical-professionals/health-policy/evidence-practice/ASPS-Rating-Scale-March-2011.pdf. Accessed July 10 2019; with permission.

Table 2	
The ASPS evidence rating scale for diagnostic studies	
Level of Evidence	**Qualifying Studies**
I	High-quality, multicentered or single-centered, cohort study validating a diagnostic test (with "gold" standard as reference) in a series of consecutive patients; or a systematic review of these studies
II	Exploratory cohort study developing diagnostic criteria (with "gold" standard as reference) in a series of consecutive patient; or a systematic review of these studies
III	Diagnostic study in nonconsecutive patients (without consistently applied "gold" standard as reference); or a systematic review of these studies
IV	Case-control study; or any of the above diagnostic studies in the absence of a universally accepted "gold" standard
V	Expert opinion developed via consensus process; case report or clinical example; or evidence based on physiology, bench research or "first principles"

From the American Society of Plastic Surgeons. Available at: https://www.plasticsurgery.org/documents/medical-professionals/health-policy/evidence-practice/ASPS-Rating-Scale-March-2011.pdf. Accessed July 10 2019; with permission.

colleagues[26] revealed that CCH (93%) resulted in more immediate transient complications compared with PNF (24%). The main limitation across these studies is applicability. For example, one trial included patients with only isolated proximal interphalangeal contractures, whereas another study excluded all patients with more than one joint disease or any patients who had received earlier treatment. Other limitations include small sample size, difficulty with blinding surgical intervention, and short follow-up duration, which limits detection of any long-term differences in recurrent disease.

Table 3	
The ASPS evidence rating scale for prognostic studies	
Level of Evidence	**Qualifying Studies**
I	High-quality, multicentered or single-centered, prospective cohort or comparative study with adequate power; or a systematic review of these studies
II	Lesser-quality prospective cohort or comparative study; retrospective cohort or comparative study; untreated controls from a randomized controlled trial; or a systematic review of these studies
III	Case-control study; or systematic review of these studies
IV	Case series with pre/posttest; or only posttest
V	Expert opinion developed via consensus process; case report or clinical example; or evidence based on physiology, bench research, or "first principles"

From the American Society of Plastic Surgeons. Available at: https://www.plasticsurgery.org/documents/medical-professionals/health-policy/evidence-practice/ASPS-Rating-Scale-March-2011.pdf. Accessed July 10 2019; with permission.

Apply to Practice

The next step of the EBP process is creating a treatment plan by integrating the best evidence found from the search, the provider's clinical expertise, and the patient's preferences and values. In this scenario, our search revealed that PNF and CCH are equally viable choices for minimally invasive treatment due to their safety and efficacy.[27–29] There was no significant difference in clinical outcomes between PNF and CCH.[26,30–32] With regard to complications, one study demonstrated increased transient complications following CCH but similar long-term follow-up.[26] These findings should be clearly presented to the patient along with discussion of risk and benefits. In any patient encounter, the best treatment plan is formed through open-communication and shared decision making by the provider and patient.

Table 4
The ASPS grade practice recommendations

Grade	Descriptor	Quality of Evidence	Implications for Practice
A	Strong recommendation	Level I evidence or consistent findings from multiple studies of levels II, III, or IV	Clinicians should follow a strong recommendation unless a clear and compelling rationale for an alternative approach is present.
B	Recommendation	Levels II, III, or IV evidence and findings are generally consistent	Generally, clinicians should follow a recommendation but should remain alert to new information and sensitive to patient preferences.
C	Option	Levels II, III, or IV evidence, but findings are inconsistent	Clinicians should be flexible in their decision making regarding appropriate practice, although they may set bounds on alternatives; patient preference should have a substantial influencing role.
D	Option	Level V: Little or no systematic empirical evidence	Clinicians should consider all options in their decision making and be alert to new published evidence that clarifies the balance of benefit vs harm; patient preference should have a substantial influencing role.

From the American Society of Plastic Surgeons. Evidence-based clinical guidelines. Available at: https://www.plasticsurgery.org/documents/medical-professionals/health-policy/evidence-practice/ASPS-Scale-for-Grading-Recommendations.pdf. Accessed July 10 2019; with permission.

Self-Evaluation

The final step to practicing evidence-based care is self-evaluation of the provider's performance. Providers should evaluate every single step of the process, starting from assessment of the patient, and identify any areas that can be improved. For example, the patient expressed preference for minimally invasive intervention but did not provide a reason why. Reasons could be attributed to complications with prior invasive procedures, unwanted postoperative outcomes, or cost. From our search, multiple investigators discussed the high cost of CCH; one article disclosed that CCH was almost 3 times more expensive than PNF.[26]

LIMITATIONS TO EVIDENCE-BASED PRACTICE AND RECOMMENDATIONS TO OVERCOME THEM

There are several limitations to practicing evidence-based care in hand surgery, such as the availability of high-quality evidence, applicability, poor critical appraisal, and insufficient resources.[6,33,34] In surgery and surgical subspecialties, RCTs can be limited by feasibility and ethical concerns. Moreover, the patients enrolled in RCTs can be nonrepresentative of patients who present to clinic, owing to factors such as age, surgical history, or comorbidities. Poor critical appraisal presents when broad search criteria or limited databases are used or there is a lack of skills and knowledge necessary to critically assess the available evidence. Last, insufficient resources, including time and cost, is a commonly cited limitation to EBP.[3,6]

To combat the lack of high-quality evidence available in surgery and hand surgery, investigators are growing the quantity and improving the quality of evidence published. From 1983 to 2003, there has been an increase in the number of published studies with control or placebo groups and RCTs in plastic surgery.[35] Similarly, there has been an increase in the number of RCTs and improvement in their methodology in hand surgery.[36] More than 400 new reviews of clinical trials are added annually to CDSR; there were 4 million downloads in 2010.[20,21] Methods to decrease the cost and time associated with practicing evidence-based care include using reliable and efficient resources, such as CDSR, and improving critical assessment proficiency and productivitiy.[2,37] Other avenues to be informed on the new literature include attending conferences, subscribing to high-quality research journals, and allocating protected research time to read and reflect on ways to improve current practice.[7,38]

DISCLOSURE

Dr. Kevin C. Chung receives funding from the National Institutes of Health and book royalties from Wolters Kluwer and Elsevier. He has received financial support from Axogen. The funding organizations had no role in the design and conduct of the study, including collection, management, analysis, and interpretation of the data. Ms. Huynh has no financial interests to declare in relation to the content of this article.

REFERENCES

1. Johnson SP, Chung KC, Waljee JF. Evidence-based education in plastic surgery. Plast Reconstr Surg 2015;136(2):258e–66e.
2. Chung KC, Swanson JA, Schmitz D, et al. Introducing evidence-based medicine to plastic and reconstructive surgery. Plast Reconstr Surg 2010;123(1):1385–9.
3. Sauerland S, Neugebauer EAM. The pros and cons of evidence-based surgery. Langenbecks Arch Surg 1999;384(5):423–31.
4. Sackett DL. Evidence-based medicine. Semin Perinatol 1997;21(1):3–5.
5. Sur R, Dahm P. History of evidence-based medicine. Indian J Urol 2011;27(4):487–9.
6. Slim K. Limits of evidence-based surgery. World J Surg 2005;29(5):606–9.
7. Sackett DL, Rosenberg WMC, Gray JM, et al. Evidence based medicine: what it is and what it isn't. BMJ 2011;312(7023):70–1.
8. Chassin MR, Galvin RW. The urgent need to improve health care quality. Institute of Medicine national roundtable. JAMA 1998;280(11):1000–5.
9. Chung KC. Evidence-based medicine: the fourth revolution in American medicine? Plast Reconstr Surg 2009;123(1):389–98.
10. Giladi AM, Chung KC. Measuring outcomes in hand surgery. Clin Plast Surg 2013;40(2):313–22.
11. Haycock C, Laser C, Keuth J, et al. Implementing evidence-based practice findings to decrease postoperative sternal wound infections. J Cardiovasc Nurs 2005;20(5):299–305.
12. Brölmann FE, Ubbink DT, Nelson EA, et al. Evidence-based decisions for local and systemic wound care. Br J Surg 2012;99(9):1172–83.
13. Gudmundsson KG, Jónsson T, Arngrímsson R. Guillaume Dupuytren and finger contractures. Lancet 2003;362(9378):165–8.
14. Shih B, Bayat A. Scientific understanding and clinical management of Dupuytren disease. Nat Rev Rheumatol 2010;6(12):715–26.
15. Lash RW, Nicholson JM, Velez L, et al. Diagnosis and management of osteoporosis. Am Fam Physician 2009;36(1):181–98.
16. Chen NC, Srinivasan RC, Shauver MJ, et al. A systematic review of outcomes of fasciotomy, aponeurotomy, and collagenase treatments for Dupuytren's contracture. Hand 2011;6(3):250–5.
17. Hurst LC, Badalamente MA, Hentz VR, et al. Injectable collagenase clostridium histolyticum for Dupuytren's contracture. N Engl J Med 2009;361(10):968–79.
18. Mcculloch P, Taylor I, Sasako M, et al. Randomised trials in surgery: problems and possible solutions. BMJ 2002;324(7351):1448–51.
19. Burns PB, Chung KC. Developing good clinical questions and finding the best evidence to answer those questions. Plast Reconstr Surg 2010;126(2):613–8.
20. Group CR. About the Cochrane Database of Systematic Reviews. Cochrane Library. Available at: http://doi.wiley.com/10.1002/14651858. Accessed July 11, 2019.
21. Bero L, Busuttil G, Farquhar C, et al. Measuring the performance of The Cochrane Library. Cochrane Library, 2012. Available at: https://www.cochranelibrary.com/cdsr/doi/10.1002/14651858.ED000048/full. Accessed July 8, 2019.
22. US National Library of Medicine. MEDLINE, PubMed and PMC (PubMed Central) - How are they different? USA.gov. Available at: https://www.nlm.nih.gov/pubs/factsheets/dif_med_pub.html%0Ahttps://www.nlm.nih.gov/bsd/difference.html. Accessed July 11, 2019.
23. Burns PB, Chung KC. The levels of evidence and their role in evidence-based medicine. Plast Reconstr Surg 2011;128(1):305–10.
24. Elsevier. Embase content. Elsevier; 2019. Available at: https://www.elsevier.com/solutions/embase-biomedical-research/embase-coverage-and-content. Accessed July 11, 2019.
25. The periodic health examination. Canadian Task Force on the Periodic Health Examination. Can Med Assoc J 1979;121(9):1193–254.
26. Skov ST, Bisgaard T, Søndergaard P, et al. Injectable collagenase versus percutaneous needle fasciotomy for Dupuytren contracture in proximal interphalangeal joints: a randomized controlled trial. J Hand Surg Am 2017;42(5):321–8.e3.
27. Eaton C. Percutaneous fasciotomy for Dupuytren's contracture. J Hand Surg Am 2011;36(5):910–5.
28. Mansha M, Flynn D, Stothard J. Safety and effectiveness of percutaneous needle fasciotomy for

Dupuytren's disease in the palm. J Hand Microsurg 2017;09(03):115–9.

29. Molenkamp S, Schouten TAM, Broekstra DC, et al. Early postoperative results of percutaneous needle fasciotomy in 451 patients with Dupuytren disease. Plast Reconstr Surg 2017;139(6):1415–21.

30. Strömberg J, Ibsen-Sörensen A, Fridén J. Comparison of treatment outcome after collagenase and needle fasciotomy for dupuytren contracture: a randomized, single-blinded, clinical trial with a 1-year follow-up. J Hand Surg Am 2016;41(9):873 80.

31. Strömberg J, Ibsen Sörensen A, Fridén J. Percutaneous needle fasciotomy versus collagenase treatment for Dupuytren contracture: a randomized controlled trial with a two-year follow-up. J Bone Joint Surg Am 2018;100(13):1079–86.

32. Nydick JA, Olliff BW, Garcia MJ, et al. A comparison of percutaneous needle fasciotomy and collagenase injection for Dupuytren disease. J Hand Surg Am 2013;38(12):2377–80.

33. Sheridan DJ, Julian DG. Achievements and limitations of evidence-based medicine. J Am Coll Cardiol 2016;68(2):204–13.

34. Sullivan KJ, Wayne C, Patey AM, et al. Barriers and facilitators to the implementation of evidence-based practice by pediatric surgeons. J Pediatr Surg 2017; 52(10):1666–73.

35. Loiselle F, Mahabir RC, Harrop AR. Levels of evidence in plastic surgery research over 20 years. Plast Reconstr Surg 2008;121(4):207–11.

36. Sugrue CM, Joyce CW, Sugrue RM, et al. Trends in the level of evidence in clinical hand surgery research. Hand 2016;11(2):211–5.

37. Chung KC, Burns PB, Davis Sears E. Outcomes research in hand surgery: where have we been and where should we go? J Hand Surg Am 2006; 31(8):1373–9.

38. Rohrich RJ. So you want to be better: the role of evidence-based medicine in plastic surgery. Plast Reconstr Surg 2010;126(4):1395–8.

Translating Hand Surgery Evidence to Policy and Practice

Jacob S. Nasser, BS[a], Kevin C. Chung, MD, MS[b],*

KEYWORDS

- Health policy • Hand surgery • Evidence-based medicine • Implementing policy
- Clinical practice guidelines

KEY POINTS

- Guidelines and policy for orthopedic and plastic surgical conditions are provided by national surgical organizations; however, hand surgery–specific guidelines are lacking.
- Conducting hand surgical outcomes research, economic analyses, evidence-based research, and basic science investigations facilitates the translation of evidence into hand surgery practice.
- Proper coordination is needed among researchers, clinicians, and policy-makers to produce evidence, implement feasible policy, and evaluate the effect of these programs.
- Institutional-level policy encourages the translation of hand surgery evidence into every-day clinical practice.
- Robust systems used to evaluate the integration of hand surgery guidelines and policy into practice is essential for the implementation of evidence-based clinical practice.

Evidence suggests that 20% of the gross domestic product in the United States will be spent on health care expenditure in 2020.[1,2] Despite the extensive spending, the performance of care remains worse than that of other high-income countries.[3] Thus, policy-makers are interested in developing initiatives to help increase the value of health care in the United States. A common way to improve patient outcomes and reduce the cost of care is the incorporation of evidence into clinical practice. For example, Fischer and Avorn[4] examined the economic implications for adherence to evidence-based recommendations for hypertension treatment and estimated that adherence-based prescribing guidelines would produce an annual savings of $1.2 billion. Nevertheless, this integration of evidence into practice requires a tenacious effort from clinicians, health policy-makers, and institutions to develop, enforce, and evaluate evidence-based policy and guidelines.

Policy and guidelines are used to inform clinicians of evidence-based recommendations by encouraging the integration of evidence into practice. However, new clinical evidence does not always influence practice immediately.[5] The integration of evidence into policy, and consequently practice, is a slow process with various challenges to implementation. For example, the United States Food and Drug Administration approved the use of intravenous tissue plasminogen activators to help ischemic stroke patients in 1996. However, it was not until 2007 when the American Heart Association and American Stroke Association established practice guidelines for the use of this treatment.[6,7] Furthermore, adherence to evidence-based guidelines is sometimes used as a performance metric. Specifically, the

a The George Washington School of Medicine and Health Sciences, Washington DC, USA; b Section of Plastic Surgery, Comprehensive Hand Center, Michigan Medicine, University of Michigan Medical School, 1500 East Medical Center Drive, 2130 Taubman Center, SPC 5340, Ann Arbor, MI 48109-5340, USA
* Corresponding author.
E-mail address: kecchung@med.umich.edu

Hand Clin 36 (2020) 145–153
https://doi.org/10.1016/j.hcl.2020.01.002

use of β-blockers is a common way to improve outcomes for patients with poor left ventricular ejection fraction. In response to evidence suggesting the underuse of this medication, medical societies, such as the American College of Cardiology and the American Heart Association, developed metrics to examine the use of β-blockers as a proxy for care performance.[8,9] Given the frequent innovations in hand surgery, enhancing the integration of guidelines and performance metrics could help provide patients with better, more uniform care.

Evidence-based practices have the potential to improve outcomes and patient satisfaction in hand surgery.[10] Reconstruction of the thumb carpometacarpal joint is one of the most common upper extremity procedures performed.[11,12] Despite the high prevalence of this surgical condition, there has been a debate regarding the optimal treatment modality since the simple complete trapeziectomy technique was discussed in 1949.[13] After the introduction of this technique, concerns of postoperative joint weakness fueled further research on other surgical procedures, such as ligament arthroplasty, to amend the disability.[14,15] Consequently, hand surgeons performed ligament arthroplasty because of the perceived benefits. Nonetheless, the most recent high-level evidence suggests that trapeziectomy is equally effective and provides a safe option for patients.[15–17] Despite this evidence, we discovered a paucity of physicians practicing simple complete trapeziectomy procedure in the United States.[15] Policy-based initiatives to implement and assess the integration of evidence into hand surgery will improve patient care in the era of value-based care.

In this article, we present a conceptual model to depict the translation of hand surgery evidence into practice and policy. Additionally, we present examples to illustrate the potential ways to develop hand surgery policy. Moreover, we apply the experiences from other medical and surgical fields in health policy to discuss recommendations for hand surgery–specific policy measures.

CONCEPTUAL MODEL

We developed a conceptual model based on the existing literature to depict how evidence regarding surgical hand conditions can be translated into policy and practice (**Fig. 1**).[5,18,19] The four components of this conceptual model include the following:

1. Synthesis and use of evidence
2. Establishment of guidelines and policy
3. Integration of policy into practice
4. Evaluation of policy and practice

The integration of evidence into clinical practice is cyclical,[20] because innovation and recent evidence require additional changes to be made to policy and practice.

Synthesis of Evidence

Researchers and clinicians can identify policies created by public and private national organizations, and meet with institutional or governmental health policy-makers to identify current issues that warrant attention.[21] For example, the Centers for Medicare & Medicaid Services developed the Hospital Readmissions Reduction Program to punish hospitals with readmission rates higher than the national average.[22] The current Hospital Readmissions Reduction Program measures performance for six medical conditions and procedures; however, researchers have investigated the feasibility of this policy for other conditions.[23] In hand surgery, we examined the emergency department use for patients after elective hand surgery because postoperative complications in hand surgery are typically more limited in severity. We apply this assessment based on existing policy but modified to establish the relevance in hand surgery.[24]

Hand surgery research comprises many different types: outcome studies, economic analyses, evidence-based studies, and basic science investigations.[25] Additionally, research on quality is focused on examining safety, effectiveness, patient-centered, timely, efficient, and equitable domains of care, as defined by the Institute of Medicine. Although a large portion of hand surgery research studies the effectiveness of particular treatment modalities, there are other components of care, such as patient-centered care, which should not be neglected when conducting research with a health policy focus.[26] For example, the Silicone Arthroplasty in Rheumatoid Arthritis (SARA) study was a long-term, multicenter prospective cohort study to compare outcomes for a surgical and nonsurgical group of rheumatoid arthritis patients. The main objective of this study was to determine the effectiveness of silicone metacarpophalangeal arthroplasty[27]; however, a secondary investigation studied the patient-centered domain of quality by examining expectations and satisfaction of the patients receiving care.[28]

Numerous hierarchies have been developed to classify scientific levels of evidence.[29] Nonetheless, the consensus among experts is that rigorous systematic reviews yield the highest level

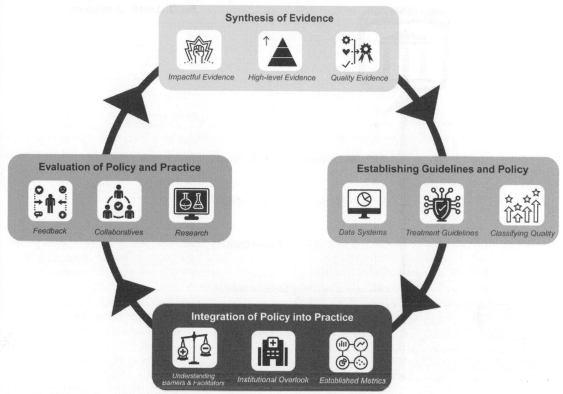

Fig. 1. Conceptual model depicting the translation of hand surgery evidence into practice and policy.

of evidence, whereas opinion-pieces and case re-ports generated the lowest level of evidence (**Fig. 2**). Although all levels of scientific evidence contribute to clinical practice, policy-makers make the greatest use out of systematic reviews because they are typically viewed as having strong evidence.[30] Sugrue and colleagues[31] investigated hand surgery articles published in six scientific journals over a 20-year period and found that although hand surgery research mir-rors that of other fields, high-quality evidence is still lacking. Hand surgery researchers can develop evidence worthy of translation into policy by applying rigorous research methodology to high-level research studies, such as systematic reviews.

Hand surgeons can apply a variety of different resources to produce high-quality, impactful research findings that influence policy. By identi-fying potential barriers before the start of a project, researchers can improve the quality of their evi-dence.[32] Numerous research guidelines exist to help encourage the production of meaningful evi-dence. The Enhancing the QUAlity and Transpar-ency Of health Research (EQUATOR) network was developed to help provide guidelines for re-searchers conducting an array of research designs.[33] For example, the Consolidated Stan-dards of Reporting Trials was developed to improve the reporting of the results derived from randomized control trials.[34] Other guidelines for economic evaluations, qualitative reports, among others are also available. Additionally, scientific journals commonly publish recommendations for improving the quality of a specific research design, which may help improve the quality of evi-dence.[35–39] For example, our research group pub-lished a guide to meta-analyses to help explain the important steps researchers should perform when synthesizing evidence using this secondary research design.[37]

Establishment of Guidelines and Policy

Establishing clinical practice guidelines and policy to enforce adherence to certain clinical practices is a process that requires extensive efforts from mul-tiple parties. The American Society of Hematology provides a general framework to depict how the development process works. This framework con-sists of eight main steps: (1) establishing a panel, (2) appointing members from a diverse range of specialties, (3) recruiting patient representatives, (4) prioritizing questions for the guideline, (5) reviewing all the available evidence, (6) developing

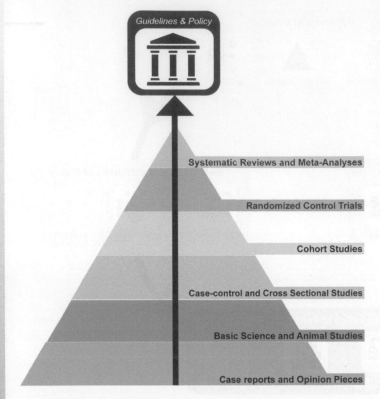

Fig. 2. Levels of evidence.

Systematic Reviews and Meta-Analyses

Randomized Control Trials

Cohort Studies

Case-control and Cross Sectional Studies

Basic Science and Animal Studies

Case reports and Opinion Pieces

Guidelines & Policy

the recommendations, (7) obtaining stakeholder and public input, and (8) submitting the final guidelines.[40] The establishment of guidelines is fluid, because the recommendations must be carefully reviewed and updated depending on new evidence and recent innovation.[41]

Numerous government agencies and national surgical societies are focused on providing surgeons with guidelines based on existing evidence to encourage the incorporation of current evidence into practice. The Agency for Healthcare Research and Quality works collaboratively with private and public organizations to comprehensively evaluate existing data on evidence in health care to help advocate for evidence-based care. Similarly, guidelines established by the American Society of Plastic Surgeons are used to develop recommendations for patient care; however, there are currently no guidelines for the treatment of hand conditions.[42] The American Association of Orthopedic Surgeons has developed clinical practice guidelines for a few surgical hand conditions to help reduce variation in carpal tunnel and distal radius fracture treatment. Additionally, a classification of the quality of evidence is provided to inform clinicians of the strength of each recommendation. The strength of the recommendations ranges from strong (highest evidence) to

consensus (no evidence).[43] Expanding guidelines for other hand conditions would facilitate the integration of evidence into hand surgery practice. Furthermore, additional information on potential interest for future research could aid clinicians to provide better evidence and recommendations.

Establishing systems to collect comprehensive data for hand surgical care will facilitate the integration of evidence into everyday practice and patient care. The Plastic Surgery Registries Network is a series of networks that collect data on plastic surgery procedures and outcomes to permit the tracking and comparison of practice performance.[44] This network has specific registries for certain plastic surgical techniques and procedures. For example, the General Registry for Autologous Fat Transfer is a United States registry to collect data on all fat grafting procedures performed in the nation. The implementation of other hand surgery–specific registries could facilitate hand surgeons on clinical decision making and identify areas of improvement.

Integration of Policy into Practice

Given the financial implications associated with adherence to evidence-based medicine, improved integration of guidelines policy into practice will aid in achieving cost savings and better value of care. Although researchers have identified best practices for the integration of evidence into medical practice, the implementation of these guidelines is difficult.[45] As pay-for-performance systems become increasingly used by private and public insurance companies,[46] institutions should determine which factors affect the translation of evidence into practice because consequences to nonadherence may influence reimbursement.

Understanding barriers and facilitators to implementation science are vital for the continued evidence-based integration.[47] Researchers have identified payment systems, information systems, physician culture, the lack of transparency in guideline development, research barriers, a lack of cooperation, and a lack of familiarity as challenges to adherence to guidelines and policy.[48] Additionally, researchers have found that evidence-based practices are encouraged by providing incentives for innovation in practice, and facilitating data transfer among health care professionals.[49,50] A summary of the various barriers and facilitators for implementing evidence-based practices in hand surgery is depicted in **Fig. 3**.[47,49,51] Although payment is considered a barrier for guideline and policy adherence, national initiatives are focused on transitioning from a volume-based to a high-value care payment model. Thus, policy-makers need to engage various stakeholders as they enforce evidence-based guidelines. Furthermore, qualitative investigations at an institutional level are imperative in overcoming the barriers that hinder evidence-based practice care, because they help identify various facilitators and barriers that occur at specific practices.

Institutions and national hand societies can facilitate the transfer of information available to hand surgeons on innovative, and recent evidence in the field by providing easy to access, convenient, and reliable resources. The AO foundation provides clinicians with educational resources for musculoskeletal injuries through various interactive and easy-to-use online programs.[52] Similar resources for hand surgical conditions may facilitate the information transfer and improve adherence to recent evidence-based findings. Moreover, promoting a clinical culture focused on collaboration, education, and research, individuals can facilitate the integration of certain guidelines into practice.

Evaluation of Policy and Practice

Although clinical practice guidelines and recommendations from medical societies are influential in guiding certain physicians, constant evaluation is needed to determine whether a particular policy is effective. The Centers for Medicare and Medicaid Services have developed 13 quality metrics for short-stay nursing home residents recovering from surgery or discharged from a short hospital stay, including the proportion of patients reporting moderate to severe pain and rate of potentially preventable hospital readmissions.[53] These metrics were developed based on an evaluation of characteristics associated with higher quality of care given during a nursing home stay. The development of specific metrics for hand surgical care may serve as a strategy to help eliminate variation in care after common hand surgeries, such as carpal tunnel or trigger finger release. Nonetheless, these metrics must be well studied before implementation. Researchers should be cognizant of the type of data used to evaluate the integration of certain guidelines and policy into practice. For example, if a surgeon is self-reporting data regarding adherence, the validity of the data may be questioned.[54] Additionally, researchers need to account for confounding variables that may influence reasons for deviation from typical practice.

Quality improvement collaboratives are becoming increasingly popular in the surgical field to help identify practice variation and improve outcomes.[55–57] For example, the Michigan Urologic Surgery Improvement Collaborative was developed in partnership with Blue Cross and Blue Shield of Michigan and Blue Care Network to improve the quality of care provided to patients with prostate cancer.[57] Because a large proportion of hand surgeries are high-volume, outpatient procedures, the success is not typically measured in terms of morbidity and mortality. Thus, measuring surgical success using quality metrics permits a more constructive report for clinicians. Our research group recently established the Michigan Collaborative Hand Initiative for Quality in Surgery (M-CHIQS). The M-CHIQS collaborative will help investigate best clinical hand surgery practices and the incorporation of evidence-based practices into medicine.

CASE STUDY: TRIGGER FINGER

Trigger finger is one of the most common hand conditions.[58] Treatment typically consists of surgical correction or corticosteroid injection.[59] Although there is a general consensus among hand surgeons regarding the types of treatment, variation exists in the number of corticosteroid injections that should be provided before the consideration of surgery. Kerrigan and Stanwix[60]

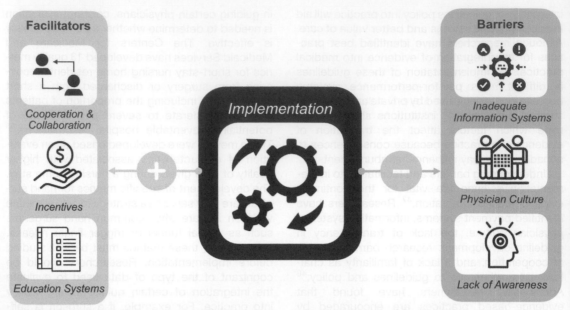

Fig. 3. Barriers and facilitators of implementing evidence-based practices in hand surgery.

conducted a cost-minimization analysis to identify the treatment algorithm that would provide the most effective results at a low cost. The authors determined that providing two injections before surgery offered adequate relief at a low cost. Amid efforts to reduce the use of wasteful resources in health care, an integration of these recommendations into practice would produce high-cost savings and improve outcomes for patients with trigger finger. Therefore, an analysis examining the adherence of a cost-effective approach to trigger finger treatment would shed light on variation in adherence and potential predictors of nonadherence. The information from such a study, in conjunction with other high-level evidence, may be useful for institutions to determine provider-level barriers that contribute to nonadherence to evidence in the literature. Additionally, information on adherence may provide hand surgery organizations incentives to produce guidelines for trigger finger treatment, given the variation in the treatment algorithm used. The identification of predictors of variation may fuel further qualitative research to identify ways to overcome barriers to implementation on a provider level. Consequently, institutional-level policies to promote the education of their clinical staff on recommendations for trigger finger treatment, in addition to other hand conditions, may be developed based on existing evidence. Furthermore, policy-based evaluations and hand surgery collaboratives, such as M-CHIQS, can provide additional data to hand surgeons regarding their adherence to established guidelines.

CASE STUDY: POSTOPERATIVE PAIN MANAGEMENT IN HAND SURGERY

Since 1999, the rate of opioid overdoses has tripled and researchers project that this rate will continue to increase.[61] Consequently, the National Institute on Drug Abuse is advocating for the use of strategies to reduce opioid consumption.[62] Although opioids offer adequate postoperative pain control, surgeons are becoming increasingly aware of the need to reduce the amount of opioid consumption after surgery, while optimizing pain relief for the patient.[63] Additionally, cost savings have been associated with a behavioral intervention to increase the use of various evidence-based strategies to manage pain in an inpatient setting.[64] Given the research on options for postoperative pain control after hand surgery, there is potential to establish guidelines and policy to reduce opioid use, improve cost savings, and improve care performance.[4] Researchers have investigated the effect of surgeon- and patient-based education to reduce the number of opioids consumed after plastic and hand surgery and found that various educational strategies are successful in reducing opioid consumption after hand surgery.[65,66] Additionally, systematic reviews revealed that individualized patient educational programs, multiple methods of education administration, and one-on-one patient education are all important in effectively educating patients postoperatively.[67] A combination of these high-level evidence studies on pain and postoperative management after hand surgery may be used to develop guidelines and policy at an institution level that focuses on educating patients on postoperative pain control and standardizing postoperative opioid prescriptions based on the surgical procedure. To implement such a policy, research at an institutional level is needed to identify cultural barriers that would prevent the integration of such policy into practice. Additionally, an established system to document the patterns of consumption and prescription after the implementation is vital to test the effects of the policy and examine provider-level factors associated with nonadherence. The system of documentation could depend on hospital billing records, to ensure the validity of the data used to evaluate the policy. Furthermore, quality collaboratives might focus on collecting data on opioid prescriptions after hand surgery.

SUMMARY

Health policy provides hand surgeons a way to take the voice of their patients and evoke a more global change. It is the role of hand surgeons, researchers, clinicians, and health care leaders of individual institutions to take an active role in the establishment of evidence and implementation of evidence into clinical practice. Using the framework provided by other medical and surgical societies, hand surgery can adopt sustainable strategies to enforce strategies that promote utmost patient care. Additionally, by advocating for state, federal, and regulatory issues that face hand surgery, individuals can impact the future of surgical hand care.

DISCLOSURE

This work was supported by a Midcareer Investigator Award in Patient-Oriented Research (2 K24-AR053120–06) to K.C. Chung. The content is solely the responsibility of the authors and does not necessarily represent the official views of the National Institutes of Health.

CONFLICTS OF INTEREST

The authors have no conflicts of interest to report.

REFERENCES

1. Shatto JD, Clemens MK. Projected Medicare expenditures under an illustrative scenario with alternative payment updates to Medicare providers. Baltimore (MD): Department of Health & Human Services, Centers for Medicare & Medicaid Services; 2011. Available at: https://www.cms.gov/research-statistics-data-and-systems/statistics-trends-and-reports/reportstrustfunds/downloads/2012tralternativescenario.pdf.
2. Keehan SP, Sisko AM, Truffer CJ, et al. National health spending projections through 2020: economic recovery and reform drive faster spending growth. Health Aff 2011;30(8):1594–605.
3. Papanicolas I, Woskie LR, Jha AK. Health care spending in the United States and other high-income countries health care spending. JAMA 2018;319(10):1024–39.
4. Fischer MA, Avorn J. Economic implications of evidence-based prescribing for hypertension: can better care cost less? Jama 2004;291(15):1850–6.
5. Glasgow RE, Green LW, Taylor MV, et al. An evidence integration triangle for aligning science with policy and practice. Am J Prev Med 2012;42(6):646–54.
6. Roth JM. Recombinant tissue plasminogen activator for the treatment of acute ischemic stroke. Proceedings-Baylor University Medical Center 2011;24(3):257–9.
7. Adams HP Jr, Del Zoppo G, Alberts MJ, et al. Guidelines for the early management of adults with ischemic stroke: a guideline from the American Heart Association/American Stroke Association Stroke Council, Clinical Cardiology Council, Cardiovascular Radiology and Intervention Council, and the Atherosclerotic Peripheral Vascular Disease and Quality of Care Outcomes in Research Interdisciplinary Working Groups: the American Academy of Neurology affirms the value of this guideline as an educational tool for neurologists. Circulation 2007;115(20):e478–534.
8. Heidenreich PA, Gholami P, Sahay A, et al. Clinical reminders attached to echocardiography reports of patients with reduced left ventricular ejection fraction increase use of β-blockers: a randomized trial. Circulation 2007;115(22):2829–34.
9. Executive summary: HFSA 2006 comprehensive heart failure practice guideline. J Card Fail 2006;12(1):10–38.
10. Zafonte B, Szabo RM. Evidence-based medicine in hand surgery: clinical applications and future direction. Hand Clin 2014;30(3):269–83.
11. Van Heest AE, Kallemeier P. Thumb carpal meta carpal arthritis. J Am Acad Orthop Surg 2008;16(3):140–51.
12. Armstrong A, Hunter J, Davis T. The prevalence of degenerative arthritis of the base of the thumb in post-menopausal women. J Hand Surg 1994;19(3):340–1.
13. Gervis WH. Excision of the trapezium for osteoarthritis of the trapezio-metacarpal joint. J Bone Joint Surg Br 1949;31(4):537–9.
14. Burton RI, Pellegrini VD. Surgical management of basal joint arthritis of the thumb. Part II. Ligament reconstruction with tendon interposition arthroplast. J Hand Surg 1986;11(3):324–32.

15. Aliu O, Davis MM, DeMonner S, et al. The influence of evidence in the surgical treatment of thumb basilar joint arthritis. Plast Reconstr Surg 2013; 131(4):816.

16. Wajon A, Vinycomb T, Carr E, et al. Surgery for thumb (trapeziometacarpal joint) osteoarthritis. Cochrane Database Syst Rev 2015;(2):CD004631.

17. Belcher H, Nicholl J. A comparison of trapeziectomy with and without ligament reconstruction and tendon interposition. J Hand Surg 2000;25(4):350–6.

18. Akobeng AK. Principles of evidence based medicine. Arch Dis Child 2005;90(8):837–40.

19. Lockwood C, Aromataris E, Munn Z. Translating evidence into policy and practice. Nurs Clin 2014; 49(4):555–66.

20. Kueny A, Shever LL, Lehan Mackin M, et al. Facilitating the implementation of evidence- based practice through contextual support and nursing leadership. J Healthc Leadersh 2015;7:29–39.

21. Pearson A, Weeks S, Stern C. Translation science and the JBI model of evidence-based healthcare. Philadelphia: Lippincott Wiliams & Wilkins; 2011.

22. Medicare CF, Services M. Readmissions reduction program (HRRP). CMS. gov; 2018. Available at: https://www.cms.gov/medicare/medicare-fee-for-service-payment/acuteinpatientpps/readmissions-reduction-program/. Accessed February 3, 2020.

23. Lucas DJ, Pawlik TM. Readmission after surgery. Adv Surg 2014;48:185–99.

24. Nasser J, Chou C-H, Chung KC. 30-day emergency department utilization after distal radius fracture treatment: identifying predictors and variation. Plast Reconstr Surg Glob Open 2019;7(9):e2416.

25. Chung KC. Clinical research in hand surgery. J Hand Surg Am 2010;35(1):109–20.

26. Epstein RM, Fiscella K, Lesser CS, et al. Why the nation needs a policy push on patient-centered health care. Health Aff 2010;29(8):1489–95.

27. Chung KC, Burns PB, Wilgis ES, et al. A multicenter clinical trial in rheumatoid arthritis comparing silicone metacarpophalangeal joint arthroplasty with medical treatment. J Hand Surg 2009;34(5): 815–23.

28. Chung KC, Nellans KW, Burns PB, et al. Patient expectations and long-term outcomes in rheumatoid arthritis patients: results from the SARA (Silicone Arthroplasty in Rheumatoid Arthritis) study. Clin Rheumatol 2015;34(4):641–51.

29. Burns PB, Rohrich RJ, Chung KC. The levels of evidence and their role in evidence-based medicine. Plast Reconstr Surg 2011;128(1):305.

30. Fox DM. Evidence of evidence-based health policy: the politics of systematic reviews in coverage decisions. Health Aff 2005;24(1):114–22.

31. Sugrue CM, Joyce CW, Sugrue RM, et al. Trends in the level of evidence in clinical hand surgery research. Hand (N Y) 2016;11(2):211–5.

32. Garas G, Ibrahim A, Ashrafian H, et al. Evidence-based surgery: barriers, solutions, and the role of evidence synthesis. World J Surg 2012;36(8): 1723–31.

33. Altman DG, Simera I, Hoey J, et al. EQUATOR: reporting guidelines for health research. Lancet 2008;371(9619):1149–50.

34. The Equator Network. 2019. Available at: https://www.equator-network.org/. Accessed April 1, 2019.

35. Shauver MS, Chung KC. A guide to qualitative research in plastic surgery. Plast Reconstr Surg 2010;126(3):1089.

36. Chung KC, Song JW, Group WS. A guide on organizing a multicenter clinical trial: the WRIST study group. Plast Reconstr Surg 2010;126(2):515.

37. Chung KC, Burns PB, Kim HM. A practical guide to meta-analysis. J Hand Surg 2006;31(10):1671–8.

38. Lau FH, Chung KC. Survey research: a primer for hand surgery. J Hand Surg 2005;30(5):893.e1-3.

39. Journal of the American Medical Association (JAMA). Research, methods, statistics. 2019. Avaliable at: https://jamanetwork.com/collections/5916/research-methods-statistics. Accessed February 3, 2020.

40. American Society of Hematology. ASH clinical practice guidelines: venous thromboembolism. 2019. Avaliable at: https://www.hematology.org/VTE/. Accessed April 11, 2019.

41. Terndrup TE. Establishing pain policies in emergency medicine. Ann Emerg Med 1996;27(4): 408–11.

42. American Society of Plastic Surgeons (ASPS). Evidence-based clinical practice guidelines. Avaliable at: https://www.plasticsurgery.org/for-medical-professionals/quality-and-registries/evidence-based-clinical-practice-guidelines. Accessed April 1, 2019.

43. American Academy of Orthopedic Surgeons. Management of carpal tunnel syndrome evidence-based clinical practice guideline. Rosemont (IL): American Academy of Orthopaedic Surgeons; 2016.

44. American Society of Plastic Surgeons (ASPS). Plastic Surgery Registries Network (PSRN). 2019. Avaliable at: https://www.plasticsurgery.org/for-medical-professionals/quality-and-registries/plastic-surgery-registries-network. Accessed April 1, 2019.

45. Tansella M, Thornicroft G. Implementation science: understanding the translation of evidence into practice. Br J Psychiatry 2009;195(4):283–5.

46. Werner RM, Kolstad JT, Stuart EA, et al. The effect of pay-for-performance in hospitals: lessons for quality improvement. Health Aff 2011;30(4):690–8.

47. Grol R, Grimshaw J. From best evidence to best practice: effective implementation of change in patients' care. Lancet 2003; 362(9391):1225–30.

48. Cabana MD, Rand CS, Powe NR, et al. Why don't physicians follow clinical practice guidelines? A framework for improvement. JAMA 1999;282(15): 1458–65.

49. NEHI. Improving physician adherence to clinical practice guidelines 2008. Available at: https://www. nehi.net/publications/53-improving-physician-adher ence-to-clinical-practice-guidelines/view.

50. Sadeghi-Bazargani H, Tabrizi JS, Azami-Aghdash S. Barriers to evidence-based medicine: a systematic review. J Eval Clin Pract 2014;20(6):793–802.

51. Cavazos J, Naik A, Woofter A, et al. Barriers to physician adherence to nonsteroidal anti-inflammatory drug guidelines: a qualitative study. Aliment Pharmacol Ther 2008;28(6):789–98.

52. AO Foundation. Curriculum development. 2019. Avaiable at: https://www.aofoundation.org/ Structure/the-ao-foundation/organization/education/ organization/Pages/Curriculum-Development.aspx. Accessed April 1, 2019.

53. Center for Medicare and Medicaid Services. Quality measures. 2019. Avaiable at: https://www.cms.gov/ medicare/quality-initiatives-patient-assessment-instruments/nursinghomequalityinits/nhqiquality-measures.html. Accessed April 9, 2019.

54. Milchak JL, Carter BL, James PA, et al. Measuring adherence to practice guidelines for the management of hypertension: an evaluation of the literature. Hypertension 2004;44(5):602–8.

55. Englesbe MJ, Dimick JB, Sonnenday CJ, et al. The Michigan Surgical Quality Collaborative: will a statewide quality improvement initiative pay for itself? Ann Surg 2007;246(6):1100–3.

56. Guillamondegui OD, Gunter OL, Hines L, et al. Using the national surgical quality improvement program and the Tennessee surgical quality collaborative to improve surgical outcomes. J Am Coll Surg 2012;214(4):709–14.

57. Montie JE, Linsell SM, Miller DC. Quality of care in urology and the Michigan Urological Surgery Improvement Collaborative. Urol Pract 2014;1(2): 74–8.

58. Blazar P, Aggarwal R. Trigger finger (stenosing flexor tenosynovitis) 2018. Available at: https://www. uptodate.com/contents/trigger-finger-stenosing-flexor-tenosynovitis?search=limited-joint-mobility-indiabetes-mellitus&selectedTitle=5~150.

59. Benson LS, Ptaszek AJ. Injection versus surgery in the treatment of trigger finger. J Hand Surg 1997; 22(1):138–44.

60. Kerrigan CL, Stanwix MG. Using evidence to minimize the cost of trigger finger care. J Hand Surg 2009;34(6):997–1005.

61. Rudd RA, Aleshire N, Zibbell JE, et al. Increases in drug and opioid overdose deaths—United States, 2000–2014. Am J Transplant 2016;16(4):1323–7.

62. National Institute on Drug Abuse. 2019. Avaiable at: https://www.drugabuse.gov/news-events/news-releases/2017/12/can-treatment-during-surgery-reduce-postoperative-opioid-use. Accessed April 11, 2019.

63. Hah JM, Bateman BT, Ratliff J, et al. Chronic opioid use after surgery: implications for perioperative management in the face of the opioid epidemic. Anesth Analg 2017;125(5):1733–40.

64. Brooks JM, Titler MG, Ardery G, et al. Effect of evidence-based acute pain management practices on inpatient costs. Health Serv Res 2009;44(1): 245–63.

65. Stanek JJ, Renslow MA, Kalliainen LK. The effect of an educational program on opioid prescription patterns in hand surgery: a quality improvement program. J Hand Surg 2015;40(2):341–6.

66. Dwyer CL, Soong M, Hunter A, et al. Prospective evaluation of an opioid reduction protocol in hand surgery. J Hand Surg 2018;43(6):516–22.e1.

67. Fredericks S, Guruge S, Sidani S, et al. Postoperative patient education: a systematic review. Clin Nurs Res 2010;19(2):144–64.

Impact of the Current United States Health Care Environment on Practice
A Private Practice Viewpoint

Walter B. McClelland Jr, MD*, Stephen M. McCollam, MD

KEYWORDS

- Private practice • Orthopedic surgery • Government regulation • Documentation burden
- Hospital consolidation • Physician burnout

KEY POINTS

- Physicians nationwide are facing increased regulatory and documentation burdens, which result in additional cost to running a medical practice.
- Private practitioners bear this burden more directly, because there are fewer providers over which to spread capital expenses or buffer losses in productivity.
- Downward financial pressures are forcing physicians to become more efficient and often result in clinical time encroaching on personal and family time in order to maintain clinical production.
- Vertical and horizontal integration of hospital systems places increased pressure on private practitioners through increased market competition.
- As the practice of medicine becomes more burdensome, physician burnout is on the rise, and changes are necessary to improve the lives of physicians.

INTRODUCTION

It is no secret that the cost of US health care has been increasing steadily year over year. As of 2017, the United States spent $10,739 per capita for health care.[1] This expenditure compares to $146 per capita in 1960. In the field of hand surgery, escalating costs have been driven by technology growth, drug development, expanded imaging options, and a sharp rise in surgical options to treat complicated and simple problems alike.

Efforts to control the unsustainable costs are increasing. Although physician salaries account for only 20% of overall health care spending,[2] decreasing reimbursement for physician services and a gradual shift of risk from insurers to health care providers have been central to cost containment strategies. At the same time, the complexity of the health care system has increased in the name of consistency and improved quality.

In many ways, the challenges faced by private practitioners in the current health care environment are similar to those employed by an academic center or private hospital system. All physicians, regardless of employment model, have encountered increased burdens related to expanding technology and regulation, increased documentation requirements, and downward financial pressures. Whereas a major health care system can spread the costs associated with these mandates across the entire network and utilize economies of scale to decrease the cost per provider, private practices have no such ability, which means each capital outlay or decrease in productivity has a direct impact on the profitability of the business.

Another key issue is the current trend of both vertical and horizontal expansion in hospital systems and academic centers. Not only are these entities hiring or purchasing practices to compete

Peachtree Orthopedics, 2001 Peachtree Road, Suite 705, Atlanta, GA 30309, USA
* Corresponding author.
E-mail address: wmcclelland@pocatlanta.com

Hand Clin 36 (2020) 155–163
https://doi.org/10.1016/j.hcl.2020.01.015
0749-0712/20/© 2020 Elsevier Inc. All rights reserved.

directly in the broad market but also they are acquiring primary care practices, urgent care centers, high school/college/professional sports coverage, and other means to control the flow of patients to their centers. As these entities reach a critical mass, they place an ever-increasing pressure on nonaffiliated practices and physicians to be either part of or intimately related to these large health care systems for both favorable contracts and access to patients.

Physicians now are required to prove their value to the health care system through a combination of high clinical success rates and low costs, which has led to a variety of poorly coordinated efforts by federal and state governments, regulatory bodies, state attorney generals, the Federal Trade Commission, the Department of Justice, state workers' compensation boards, hospital systems, and medical insurance companies to prove health care dollars are being spent wisely. When combined with a confluence of other unrelated socioeconomic and litigation trends, these regulations have created unprecedented challenges to private practice physicians who deliver the majority of care to patients in the United States.

The authors see these challenges as falling into 4 categories that are summarized: growing technology and regulatory burden, growing provider documentation burden, downward financial pressures, and increased market competition.

GROWING TECHNOLOGY/REGULATORY BURDEN

In recent years, the government has progressively mandated a series of technological upgrades in health care. Although the rationale behind these upgrades has been an attempt to improve quality of care, standardization of patient experience, and interconnectedness of the health care system, all of these have occurred at the expense of physician practices. In addition, some mandates transfer additional risk to the physician, both in terms of financial liability if certain processes are not met and of legal liability if patient resources are not provided.

Mandated Use of Electronic Medical Record

In the Centers for Medicare & Medicaid Services (CMS) 2019 quality reporting program, 25% to 30% of the Merit-based Incentive Payment System (MIPS) score[3] is predicated on the use of an electronic medical record (EMR) that allows for exchange of privacy-protected clinical information with patients on an approved portal, electronic prescribing of medications, electronic transfer of health records to referring physicians, receiving

and storage of new health information (imaging reports, laboratory data, and therapy progress notes), clinical data registry reporting, and other tasks, such as immunization registry reporting.

The purchase and implantation of an EMR are expensive and time consuming. The capital outlay required to obtain and integrate one of these systems results in a direct increase in business costs and reciprocal loss in net revenue. In addition, the workflow of most EMRs is more cumbersome than focused record keeping, resulting in longer work hours and/or a reduced number of patients seen per day. This workflow burden results in a temporary (if not permanent) loss of productivity, which also can result in lower revenue to the medical group.

EHR purchase and implementation is burdensome particularly on small groups or solo practices that cannot pool resources and spread costs like larger practices. There also is considerable risk in choosing the right EMR, because certain products have failed to succeed, and others have consolidated or been acquired.

Increased Focus on Quality of Care

As the health care paradigm has shifted from volume to value,[4] physicians have been saddled with additional burdens to demonstrate the high quality of the care they provide. This mandate comes in the form of reporting metrics that the medical practice must take the time to collect and submit at the requested intervals. As lawmakers debate the best way to define and measure value, these metrics are adjusted, and the physician practice has to adjust accordingly (eg, the 2017 transition from Physician Quality Reporting System to MIPS). In preparation for more stringent assessments of value that may be forthcoming, some practices have employed third-party patient outcomes programs to prospectively collect outcomes data that ultimately could be used to demonstrate quality of care. All these programs require additional time, staff, and cost to physician practices.

Changes in Reimbursement to Incentivize Use of in Office Digital Radiography

Beginning in 2017, Medicare reimbursements for the technical component for outpatient radiography were reduced by 20% for film-based radiographs. For computed radiography, the initial reduction was 7%, increasing to 10% by 2023.[5]

Although digital radiography (DR) results in lower radiation exposure, the purchase and implantation of DR equipment are expensive and may not be cost effective for lower-volume providers that cannot appreciate the faster imaging time per patient. This is true especially for small group practices and solo practitioners.

Federally Mandated Translation Services for Non–english-speaking Patients

Numerous state and federal laws have evolved to require the use of translation services and written translated materials for non–English-speaking, deaf, and hard-of-hearing patients.[6] These laws date back to Civil Rights Act of 1964 and have been fortified with the Americans with Disabilities Act implemented in 1990 and the updated Affordable Care Act (ACA) of 2016. There also is supporting state law in all 50 states requiring these services.

This altruistic mandate undoubtedly provides enhanced care to language-deficient and hearing-deficient patients. However, setting up protocols and thresholds for use for translation services can be complicated and costly in terms of disrupted workflow in the office and operating room setting.

Increased Privacy Requirements in Health Insurance Portability and Accountability Act Laws

The training of staff and physicians to grasp the complexities of the Health Insurance Portability and Accountability Act laws and create new protocols requires lots of time and continuous training modules for annual updates.[7] Texting radiographs or clinical pictures on cell phones has been discouraged, unless certain protocols or encryption software is utilized. These burdens can delay or prevent spontaneous collaboration between colleagues used to improve care.[8]

Increased Risk of Hacking and Cybercrime

The risk of data breach and malicious hacking is rampant across the consumer sector. Relevant to the medical industry, protected health information (PHI) has been deemed far more valuable on the dark Web than credit card data. Groups must employ information technology experts and invest in appropriate safety mechanisms to protect the vast amounts of PHI stored on practice servers. Threats of hacking, malware, and phishing are ever-changing, requiring a continual investment in time and resources to stay clear of harm.

If PHI is obtained inappropriately, then groups could find themselves faced with ransom demands, legal fees, or government penalties as part of the fallout. Several years ago, several orthopedic practices were hacked by a group calling themselves the Dark Lord, who demanded ransom to buy back stolen data from these groups' computer servers. Several class action suits were filed as a result and are still winding their way through the appellate courts in Georgia. As awareness of this risk grows, many groups are spending additional money to invest in data breach insurance policies.

Increased Educational and Compliance Burden Associated with the Opioid Crisis

The opioid crisis has resulted in many mandated training sessions for doctors and other providers. Three hours of opioid-specific CME are now required for renewal of state licensure in Georgia. There are ongoing negotiations at the Georgia State Board of Workers' Compensation to create mandated formularies for opioid prescribing. Many states have initiated a prescription drug monitoring program (PDMP), which providers much check before prescribing opioids and other restricted drugs and then document that they consulted the PDMP with each script dispensed. Although well intentioned, this program also creates a drag on workflow, resulting in more unit time spent with each patient, translating into longer work days or fewer patients seen, both of which can affect practice revenue adversely, either in increased overtime pay for employees or reduced patients treated per day.

Mandatory Conversion from International Classification of Diseases, Ninth Revision, to International Classification of Diseases, Tenth Revision

The *International Classification of Diseases, Version 9*, had been used for many years for all diagnostic coding. On October 1, 2015, the federal government mandated providers to convert to *International Classification of Diseases, Version 10*. This mandate resulted in the need to document laterality and more specificity in diagnoses. Increasing the sheer number and complexity of orthopedic diagnoses resulted in coding challenges for providers.[9,10] Many hours of training were required to comply with this mandate. Although crosswalking software is a component of many EMRs, the workflow to properly document a given diagnosis is now more time consuming, resulting in inefficiencies and increased time spent with coding. It also increases opportunities for incorrect coding, which can result in payment delays or increased denials as insurance companies identify inconsistencies in the medical record.

Outdated Stark Laws

The Stark laws of the 1990s were established to prevent health care fraud and abuse.[11] Specifically, the laws prohibited the referral of patients paid for by Medicare to any entity in which the provider has a financial relationship. Certain in-office ancillary exemptions were established, including in-office physical and occupational therapy and in-office imaging services (radiographs, magnetic resonance imaging, computed tomography, and ultrasound). Physician-owned ambulatory surgery centers also were exempted, as long as profitability for patients insured through federal insurance programs was not assigned based on patent volume.

Since the inception of the Stark laws, numerous federal legislative and regulatory mandates[12] (eg, Medicare Access and CHIP Reauthorization Act of 2015 [MACRA] laws) have incentivized the creation of joint ventures between physicians and other entities (such as hospitals) to improve the quality of patient care. Unfortunately, the current Stark laws do not easily allow for such partnerships to be created. Efforts to modernize the Stark laws have stalled in Congress. This inability for physicians to financially partner with hospitals and other health care entities creates barriers to appropriate population management of high-risk groups with chronic diseases, such as diabetes and hypertension.

GROWING DOCUMENTATION BURDEN

As an extension of the focus on cost containment, there has been increased scrutiny and criticism of physician documentation. Physicians now are held to a higher standard to justify their level of coding, and insurance carriers are using incidents of incomplete/inadequate coding or inconsistencies in the medical record as rationale for underpayment or payment denials. More time spent on documentation and coding means either less productivity, because providers are unable to see the same number of patients they could previously, or additional time spent after hours to complete the documentation burden, which detracts from personal and family time and directly contributes to physician burnout.

Increasing Documentation Burden for Office Visits

With the advent of the Documentation Guidelines for Evaluation and Management Services in 1995, physicians have been obligated to satisfy a certain number of bullet points within the categories of history, physical examination, and medical decision making to justify their level of evaluation and management billing. These data points must be presented clearly in the documentation or risk reduced or refused payments from insurers for services rendered.

Practices either must hire more staff or outsource these services to third-party vendors to combat denials and clawbacks and mitigate lost reimbursement. Although most current EMR systems offer features to standardize notes based on the level of complexity, they require additional financial investment and additional time to create templates and typically produce a note that is cumbersome and difficult to interpret. The additional time required to meet these documentation thresholds takes up time that could be used for other work activities or spent for personal/family endeavors.

Increased Insurer Reliance on Utilization Review

Utilization management is defined as "the evaluation of the medical necessity, appropriateness and efficient use of health care services, procedures and facilities under the provisions of the patient's health benefits plan."[13] In theory, this concept is designed as a tool to maintain quality control and cost containment in health care. In practice, it has become a time-consuming and frustrating impediment to the independent practice of medicine.

Insurers are relying to a greater and greater degree on protocols, algorithms, and checklists to determine when diagnostic and surgical services are indicated. Sometimes these guidelines are based on specialty-specific appropriate use criteria, but at other times they seem to be an arbitrary creation of the insurer, without solid basis in clinical science. Reviews often are performed by nurses, with the final judgment made by physicians who may or may not be trained in the specialty of interest. In all cases, these judgements are made by individuals who have not spoken to or examined the patient.

Hand surgeons are affected more frequently than other specialties because the surgical procedures and advanced imaging studies typically are on the more expensive side, and curtailing these interventions can have a larger impact on an insurer's bottom line. Peer-to-peer discussions are time consuming, inconvenient, and often frustrating interactions. Physicians either must handle these themselves above and beyond their baseline clinical duties or employ their staff to do so, which detracts from other clinical and administrative duties. In a 2016 American Medical Association

(AMA) survey, 75% of physicians described the burden of prior authorization to be high or extremely high.[14]

In the authors' experience, peer-to-peer appeals often are successful, because most physicians have sound logic for their treatment recommendations, making the process of completing the peer-to-peer appeal even more frustrating, because the end result typically is proceeding with the plan as it initially was outlined. Those appeals handled by physician assistants or staff members seem to have a lower success rate, which places physicians in an awkward position of deciding whether to handle the majority of these themselves or risk having the care of their patients interrupted.

Ever-Changing Requirements by Insurers Before Issuing Payment for Services Rendered

Insurance companies are in the enviable position of being able to dictate terms to physician practices on what they require before providing payment for services rendered. In many cases, these requirements are determined unilaterally and provided via a courtesy update so physician practices know what is expected. In some cases, however, these requirements are not overtly stated, and it takes a physician practice to identify trends in denials in order to decipher what is expected. These expectations rarely are uniform across payers, which means additional experience and knowledge are required to navigate each Insurance company successfully.

Prepayment audit reviews are an entity in which a physician is flagged by an insurer based on billing volume or coding techniques that fall outside the norm for the specialty and geographic area.[15] Once this occurs, a provider's claims may be denied on receipt by the insurer, with a request for all documentation to be provided for review before a determination on payability can be made. Not only does this submit the provider to further scrutiny and risk decreasing reimbursement but also it delays payments of the claim substantially.

The overall result is a feeling of a moving target, where physician practices feel as though the rules are always changing. Although insurance companies argue these requirements are designed to maintain quality and limit unnecessary expense to the health care system, the obvious supposition on behalf of physicians is that these rules are designed to justify nonpayment or reduced payment for physician services. In many cases, it feels as though the insurance companies are hoping providers either will give up out of frustration or see the potential gains as not worth the financial and time investment needed.

DOWNWARD FINANCIAL PRESSURE

Although physician salaries represent only a small portion of overall health care spending, policy makers and insurance companies have seen physician compensation as a key area for cost containment. Because physicians historically have been a poorly organized labor group, with inadequate attention and resources dedicated to advocacy, reimbursement rates have seen a slow decline in many areas, forcing physicians to maximize efficiency, making up for the decrease in unit revenue with an increase in volume. Decreased reimbursement has also forced practitioners to engage in alternative payment models, where an increased share of the financial risk is shifted from the insurer to the provider.

Decreasing Reimbursement per Unit Work by Benchmarking Off Medicare

In the 1990s, commercial insurers began benchmarking their reimbursement rates to Medicare. In inflation-adjusted dollars, the commercial rates have experienced a downward trend with inadequate cost of living adjustments despite underfunded mandates for technology upgrades, such as DR and EMRs.

Risk of Recovery Audit Contractors Audits, Clawbacks, and Penalties from Federally Funded Health Programs

Recovery Audit Contractors were allowed to evaluate improper Medicare payments to providers retrospectively beginning with a pilot program formulated in 2003.[16,17] If documentation requirements are not met, then penalties and clawbacks can be assessed. Numerous group medical practices have been assessed large fines, which can be disputed only through an appeals process or litigation. Internal compliance programs have become necessary for medical groups to avoid specific providers placing the financial well-being of the group at risk, resulting in business office costs and increased overhead.

Lack of Advanced Payment Model Opportunities Within the Centers for Medicare & Medicaid Services Quality Reporting Program

The 2015 landmark MACRA legislation[18] created what has come to be known as the quality reporting program for most Medicare provider participants. Two participation tracks have been designated: MIPS and the Advanced Alternative Payments Model (APM). Reporting requirements for MIPS have 4 components—quality, promoting interoperability, improvement activities, and cost—that are subject to annual changes in weighting to arrive at an overall performance score. This score then is used to adjust payments 2 years after the reporting period.[18] Criticisms of this program are numerous, which include its complexity, reporting burden, inconsistent weighting of the components from year to year, and the 2-year delay in reporting and payment adjustments.[19]

The annual cost of living update for MIPS is 0.25% and for APM is 0.75%, substantially below the annual rate of inflation, which results in a net decline in the annually adjusted reimbursement rate. As it currently stands, the annual payment updates drop to zero in 2020. Additional annual payment bonuses of up to 5% are available for APM participants. Currently, there are no APM opportunities for hand surgeons and many other specialists. This unbalanced incentive payment system, along with the imminent loss of annual cost of living increases and no access to APMs, creates a no-win scenario, with decreasing annual reimbursement while the burden of reporting these quality measures remains on the physician.

Unbalanced Negotiating Options as a Legacy Effect of the McCarran-Ferguson Act

The McCarran-Ferguson act of 1945 gave protections to the burgeoning health insurance industry by allowing state regulatory law to preempt federal law, creating a complex set of rules to prevent physicians from sharing business-related contract information between group practices. Although insurers know what the market rate is for insurance contracts, physician groups do not, making it impossible to demand equal financial reimbursement across local, regional, or national markets. As a response, some physician groups have pursued membership in physician-hospital organizations to allow for improved market leverage on contracted hospital and group medical practice rates.

Unilateral Downcoding of Charges

At times, payers, such as state workers' compensation boards, federal programs, and private insurers, have decided unilaterally to decrease reimbursement rates or pay only a percentage of billed charges for a given service. With a complex and time-consuming appeal process, pursuing correction of these underpayments often is not a cost-effective undertaking for medical practices, resulting in a net loss of revenue through incremental reduction of payments.

INCREASED MARKET COMPETITION

Private practitioners have seen an increase in competition in a variety of ways in recent years. As awareness has increased that orthopedic surgery is a highly lucrative specialty, there has been an equal increase in those attempting to control care of the musculoskeletal patient, ranging from hospital systems to other specialists. This increase, in combination with certain regulatory issues, has forced orthopedists to fight even harder to distinguish themselves in the marketplace.

Private practitioners have to make a particular effort to stand out, because there is not the same infrastructure in place for patient referrals as exists for those in an academic or hospital-employment models, resulting in more financial expenditure (eg, increased marketing expense), more effort above and beyond normal clinical obligations (eg, managing social media and participating in community events), and more catering to patient schedules that may detract from a physician's family and personal time (eg, after-hours clinics).

Horizontal and Vertical Integration of Hospital Systems and Academic Centers

The orthopedic market in Atlanta, as in many major metropolitan areas, is in the midst of a massive consolidation of health care services. Hospital systems are rapidly buying up smaller independent facilities and placing them under their umbrella, leading to fewer players in the market, with each wielding more clout, controlling more resources, and exerting pressure over a larger geographic footprint.

In addition to this horizontal expansion, hospital systems are engaging in vertical integration as well. By acquiring primary care groups, therapy services, urgent care centers, imaging services, and high school/college/professional sports affiliations, these systems are attempting to direct patients into their network and keep them there through their course of treatment. Because private practitioners often do not have access to these feeder networks, there is fear that patient volume will be inadequate to support their businesses over the long term.

In the orthopedic market, private practitioners typically have provided specialty services to the hospital system in a collegial partnership. In the current environment, hospitals frequently threaten private practices that they should either sell their practice to the hospital or engage in a close business relationship (like a professional services agreement) or else expect heightened competition as the hospital hires their own orthopedic staff.

Mergers of Major Health Care Insurers

Like hospital systems, there also has been merger activity among private health insurers. Although some of these in recent years have been unsuccessful—such as Aetna/Humana and Anthem/Cigna—others have failed, resulting in fewer overall payers, with each representing a larger percentage of the population. Thus, all providers are put in a weakened negotiating position with contracts, in particular, smaller private groups that represent a smaller number of providers.

Certificate of Need Laws and Moratorium on Physician-Owned Hospitals

The Certificate of Need (CON) programs emerged at the state level after a federal mandate that was part of the 1974 federal Health Planning Resources Development Act. This mandate was repealed in 1987, and the status of CON has been in flux since that time, with 12 states repealing the laws altogether and others making modifications.[20] In Georgia, current CON laws favor the hospital systems, because their considerable lobbying efforts have succeeded in blocking multiple privately funded projects.

As part of the 2010 ACA, the government placed a moratorium on physician-owned hospitals. These facilities have been shown to provide lower cost care with good patient outcomes, low complication rates, high patient satisfaction, and high physician satisfaction.[21] Incentivizing physicians financially has proved to have a strong impact on delivering high-quality and cost-effective care.

These CON and ACA regulations limit physician-led innovation and exist largely because of the strong hospital lobby. As the data supporting physician-led ventures increase, there will be a need to reconsider their role in today's health care system.

Scope of Practice Encroachment

The field of orthopedics currently is involved in several turf wars, as other specialties attempt to encroach on its historic scope of practice. Podiatrists are attempting to treat pathology extending proximally to the tibial tubercle. Chiropractors are engaging in injection therapies and other nonsurgical modalities. Physiatrists now are performing regenerative medicine and minimally invasive surgical procedures, such as carpal tunnel releases. In the state of Georgia, physical therapists now are allowed to treat patients for 21 days or 8 visits before obtaining a physician referral.[22] All these issues decrease the market share of orthopedic surgeons, as other providers attempt to infringe on treatment of musculoskeletal issues.

SUMMARY

Over the past few years, there has been an increasing awareness that the confluence of the factors, discussed previously, has taken a significant toll on the medical community, especially in medical groups that lack the size and scale to respond to the mandated infrastructure investment upgrades. With increasing cost of doing business, decreasing reimbursement for services rendered, and increased documentation and administrative burdens, it is a difficult time to practice medicine, particularly in the private practice sphere.

Although the business impact of these factors has contributed to more and more physicians retiring or becoming employed by large health care entities, the personal impact cannot be overlooked. Physician burnout is now a well-recognized issue affecting medicine overall, resulting in emotional exhaustion, depersonalization, and reduced personal accomplishment.[23] Numerous major medical organizations, including the CMS, state medical societies, physician specialty organizations, hospitals, and the AMA, are focusing on the causes and impact burnout has on their members.

The American Society for Surgery of the Hand (ASSH) made physician burnout a mega issue to be studied by a subgroup of the Young Leaders Program. Based on the findings and recommendations of this group, the ASSH has convened a task force to study the issue further and determine what steps the organization can take to curtail and address this rising problem.

Efforts to address these issues have begun in earnest. The CMS has proposed decreasing the documentation requirements for office visits, except for the most complex of patients. The AMA, American Academy of Orthopaedic Surgeons, American College of Surgeons, and other specialty organizations have submitted constructive comments during the public comment period offered by the CMS. Work groups have been established by the AMA to work with the CMS on these suggested documentation reductions.

Several medical organizations, such as the AMA, have created Web-based learning modules to educate physician members on how to identify signs and symptoms of burnout as well as tools to improve physician workflow burdens. Hospital systems are dedicating increased resources to helping physicians identify symptoms and address causes of burnout. It has been widely recognized that if the commitment, health, and enthusiasm of today's medical workforce cannot be maintained, then the entire system is in jeopardy.

Although many challenges exist in maintaining a successful private practice in today's health care market, there still are innumerable benefits to this practice model. Those committed to independent practice appreciate the involvement in critical decision making, the collegial atmosphere that accompanies a smaller business, the entrepreneurial atmosphere, and the opportunity for financial gain based on one's own hard work. As efforts progress to counteract some of the professional challenges, outlined previously, the authors feel this existence of a private practitioner will continue to improve.

DISCLOSURE

The authors have nothing to disclose.

REFERENCES

1. Centers for Medicare and Medicaid Services. National health expenditure data. 2019. Available at: https://www.cms.gov/Research-Statistics-Data-and-Systems/Statistics-Trends-and-Reports/NationalHealthExpendData/NationalHealthAccountsHistorical.html. Accessed November 11, 2019.

2. Price G, Norbeck T. Debunking myths: physicians' incomes are too high and they are the cause of rising health care costs. In: Forbes. 2017. Available at: https://www.forbes.com/sites/physiciansfoundation/2017/11/27/debunking-myths-physicians-incomes-are-too-high-and-they-are-the-cause-of-rising-health-care-costs/#1b226db11400. Accessed November 18, 2019.

3. Centers for Medicare and Medicaid Services. Quality measurement methodology and resources. CMS; 2019.

4. Porter ME, Lee TH. From volume to value in health care: the work begins. JAMA 2016;316(10):1047–8.

5. Dent CW. 114th congress (2015-2016): consolidated appropriations act, 2016. 2015. Available at: https://www.congress.gov/bill/114th-congress/house-bill/2029/text. Accessed September 1, 2019.

6. Chen AH, Youdelman MK, Brooks J. The legal framework for language access in healthcare settings: title VI and beyond. J Gen Intern Med 2007; 22(Suppl 2):362–7.

7. Division (DCD) DC. HHS seeks public input on improving care coordination and reducing the regulatory burdens of the HIPAA rules. HHS.gov. 2018. Available at: https://www.hhs.gov/about/news/2018/12/12/hhs-seeks-public-input-improving-care-coordination-and-reducing-regulatory-burdens-hipaa-rules.html. Accessed September 1, 2019.

8. Is Texting in Violation of HIPAA? HIPAA Journal. Available at: https://www.hipaajournal.com/texting-violation-hipaa/. Accessed September 1, 2019.

9. Caskey RN, Abutahoun A, Polick A, et al. Transition to international classification of disease version 10, clinical modification: the impact on internal medicine and internal medicine subspecialties. BMC Health Serv Res 2018;18(1):328.

10. Krive J, Patel M, Gehm L, et al. The complexity and challenges of the International Classification of Diseases, Ninth Revision, Clinical Modification to International Classification of Diseases, 10th Revision, Clinical Modification transition in EDs. Am J Emerg Med 2015;33(5):713–8.

11. Social Security Administration O. Compilation of the social security laws: limitation on certain physician referrals. Available at: https://www.ssa.gov/OP_Home/ssact/title18/1877.htm. Accessed September 20, 2019.

12. Centers for Medicare & Medicaid Services (CMS), HHS. Medicare Program; Merit-Based Incentive Payment System (MIPS) and Alternative Payment Model (APM) Incentive Under the Physician Fee Schedule, and Criteria for Physician-Focused Payment Models. Final rule with comment period. Fed Regist 2016;81(214):77008–831.

13. Akosa AN. Precertification, denials and appeals: reducing the hassles. Fam Pract Manag 2006; 13(6):45–8.

14. American Medical Association. 2016 AMA prior authorization physician survey. Available at: https://www.ama-assn.org/sites/ama-assn.org/files/corp/media-browser/public/government/advocacy/2016-pa-survey-results.pdf. Accessed October 22, 2019.

15. Levy MJ, Marder SL. Understanding prepayment audit reviews. Available at: https://weisszarett.com/index.aspx?TypeContent=CUSTOMPAGEARTICLE&custom_pages_articlesID=15702#_ftn2. Accessed December 2, 2019.

16. Council for Medicare Integrity. A History of the RAC Program. Available at: http://medicareintegrity.org/wp-content/uploads/2015/02/RAC_Timeline_v4.pdf. Accessed December 4, 2019.

17. Centers for Medicare and Medicaid services. Program History and Authorities. 2017. Available at: https://www.cms.gov/Research-Statistics-Data-and-Systems/Monitoring-Programs/recovery-audit-program-parts-c-and-d/Program-History-and-Authorities.html. Accessed September 1, 2019.

18. Burgess MC. House - Energy and Commerce; Ways and Means; Judiciary; Agriculture; Natural Resources; Budget. Medicare Access and CHIP Reauthorization Act of 2015. 2015. Available at: https://www.congress.gov/bill/114th-congress/house-bill/2/text. Accessed September 1, 2019.

19. Crosson FJ, Christianson JB, Bricker A, et al. Medicare Payment Advisory Commission. 2018:468.

20. National Conference of State Legislatures. CON - Certificate of need state laws. Available at: http://www.ncsl.org/research/health/con-certificate-of-need-state-laws.aspx. Accessed December 14, 2019.

21. Shute D. Is it time to lift the ban on physician owned hospitals? Med Econ 2018;96(9). Available at: https://www.medicaleconomics.com/business/it-time-lift-ban-physician-owned-hospitals. Accessed October 11, 2019.

22. American Physical Therapy Association. Level of patient access to physical therapist services in the US. 2019. Available at: https://www.apta.org/uploadedFiles/APTAorg/Advocacy/State/Issues/Direct_Access/DirectAccessbyState.pdf. Accessed November 22, 2019.

23. Maslach C, Jackson SE, Leiter MP. Maslach burnout inventory. 3rd edition. Palo Alto (CA): Consulting Psychologists Press; 1996.

The Influence of the United States Health Care Environment and Reform on Academic Medical Centers

Lars Matkin, MD, MBA[a], David Ring, MD, PhD[b],*

KEYWORDS

- Academic medical center • Affordable care act • Health policy • Accountable care organizations

KEY POINTS

- Passage of the Affordable Care Act greatly influenced payer mix at academic medical centers.
- Academic medical centers have had mixed results with alternative payment models and continue to struggle to adapt to changes in policy.
- Academic medical centers are increasingly required to compete with large private health care systems.
- Uncertainty in the future of health care policy has significant influence on the future of academic medical centers.

INTRODUCTION

In 2010, the Affordable Care Act (ACA) was signed into law. It is the largest single piece of health care legislation since the Social Security Amendments of 1965, which created the Medicare and Medicaid programs. The ACA was intended to expand insurance coverage by implementing an individual mandate, requiring all US citizens to either purchase health insurance or be subject to a tax. It also provided federal funds to expand Medicare and established government-run health care exchanges whereby insurance could be purchased with assistance from federal subsidies. With the choice to accept the Medicaid expansion and set up state run exchanges left to individual states, there remains variability in the implementation and coverage of individuals in each state.

Incorporated into the law were numerous measures to shift the focus of health care to a value-based reimbursement system. Value based care was further advanced with the Medicare Access and CHIP reauthorization Act of 2015 (MACRA), which implemented provider reimbursement incentives focused on value through the merit-based incentive system (MIPS), while also encouraging the development of alternative practice models.

Since its signing, the ACA has come under numerous legal and political challenges, including Supreme Court rulings and changes under the Trump Administration, softening or eliminating aspects of the law. These changes, and the continued volatility of the future of health care in the United States, will affect academic medical centers (AMCs) and their associated practices as they try to remain competitive and current while maintaining their focus on excellence and education.

ACADEMIC MEDICAL CENTERS

AMCs may be especially vulnerable to changes in how we pay for health care. There are approximately 350 AMCs across the United States, most

a Orthopedic Surgery Department, University of Texas at Austin, Health Discovery Building HDB 6.706, 1701 Trinity Street, Austin, TX 78712, USA; b Department of Surgery and Perioperative Care, University of Texas at Austin, Health Discovery Building HDB 6.706, 1701 Trinity Street, Austin, TX 78712, USA
* Corresponding author.
E-mail address: David.Ring@austin.utexas.edu

Hand Clin 36 (2020) 165–169
https://doi.org/10.1016/j.hcl.2020.01.003

located in major metropolitan areas. They tend to be large, nonprofit, acute care facilities (median of 477 staffed beds).[1] In addition to caring for complex and socioeconomically diverse patients, AMCs also have a focus on research and education. This focus results in a complex financial and operational structure, with high fixed costs and high disease severity and case complexity. These diverse demands can increase costs, administrative burden, and the use of complex cost sharing to support institutional goals.

Many AMCs provide a large proportion of care for the underinsured and uninsured and are designated as safety net hospitals, meaning they care for all patients regardless of insurance or ability to pay. To offset costs, disproportionate share hospital programs and other compensation methods provide financing to hospitals with safety net status with most funds going to AMCs.[2] AMCs also receive other financial incentives to offset teaching costs, including Indirect Medical Education payments, which provide additional reimbursement per case based on the number of residents an institution employs.[3] AMCs also tend to have higher reimbursements because of higher diagnostic-related group weights assigned to each episode of care on more medically complex patients. AMCs also frequently have more complex cases, resulting in higher reimbursements.[4]

The central location of AMCs in or near urban centers increases costs and places them closer to higher concentrations of homeless and indigent people. These patients also tend to have more severe health care issues, resulting in a higher case mix index, a weighted index representing higher clinically complex and resource-intensive caseloads.[5,6] The suburbanization of the American working class starting in the 1950s further exacerbates this imbalanced payer mix as working, privately insured families moved out of the traditional catchment areas of AMCs, while increasing the proportion of younger patients who are more likely to be uninsured.[7]

AMCs also have some characteristics that can buffer financial stressors and position them to lead innovation in health care and in the development of new care models. The overall size and expense of AMCs care coverage allow them to control all aspects of treatment, from primary to quaternary care. Nonprofit status and the long-term financial outlook allow them to make longer-term investments and cost shift to accommodate expenditures that for-profit institutions may not be able to achieve. AMCs also attract providers involved in research and innovation,

potentially enhancing the expertise needed to develop alternative care models. Also, because of the high cost and lower productivity associated with teaching institutions, AMCs are more likely to use salaried payment models for providers, resulting in compensation that is not directly linked to productivity, easing transitions away from fee-for-service compensation.[8]

THE CHANGING PAYER MIX FOR ACADEMIC MEDICAL CENTERS

The ACA increased the proportion of Americans with insurance by expanding Medicaid to patients who make less than 138% of the federal poverty level. The law mandated that each state accept a portion of the cost, reaching 10% by 2020.[9] However, in 2012, the Supreme Court ruled that individual states must have the ability to accept the expansion, allowing state governments to choose to either accept federal funding to expand Medicaid or continue existing programs. This created a "coverage gap" for patients who did not qualify for Medicaid or federal subsidies in states that did not expand their Medicaid programs.[10] As of 2019, 33 states have accepted the expansion. Uninsured rates in states that did not expand Medicaid have remained significantly higher than expansion states with an average of 14.1% versus 7.3% in 2016.[11]

The ACA also attempted to incentivize individuals who do not qualify for Medicare to get health insurance by creating an individual mandate paired with income-based subsidies that could be used on federal health care exchanges.[12,13] These changes were effective in reducing the uninsured population from 44 million (15%) to 27 million (9%) between 2008 and 2017.[14] The reduction in uninsured patients has significantly affected AMCs, with the proportion of patients presenting to emergency rooms and safety net clinics with insurance increasing significantly since the expansion.[7,15,16] This change in coverage has resulted in decreased uncompensated care costs, increased Medicaid revenue, and an overall improvement in margins for affected hospitals.[17]

Before the ACA, there had been other efforts to reduce uninsured populations in the United States. For example, in 2006, Massachusetts implemented universal coverage for Massachusetts residents. This universal coverage reduced the uninsured rate of patients treated for traumatic injury by 40%.[18] This reform resulted in fewer patients forgoing care because of cost and more patients having a personal doctor. It was also found to have a greater effect on socioeconomically disadvantaged patients.[19]

ALTERNATIVE PAYMENT MODELS FOR ACADEMIC MEDICAL CENTERS

Built into the ACA were incentives for the development of alternative payment models (APMs) and other value-based initiatives. This included the establishment of the Medicare Shared Savings Program (MSSP), which incentivized the formation of Accountable Care Organizations (ACO). These organizations provided comprehensive care to a defined population of patients and stand to share any cost savings (or losses) provided by reducing unnecessary spending and improving care. Also included in the ACA was the development of the Center for Medicare and Medicaid Innovation. With the passing of MACRA in 2015, further incentives emerged focusing on value and APMs through MIPS, which imposed bonuses or penalties to providers based on their ability to meet specific goals in care.

AMCs became some of the first centers to attempt the accountable care model. AMCs already had well-coordinated care systems that included most major components of treatment, including both primary and specialty care. They also have the ability to accept higher levels of risk and maintain a longer-term financial outlook as nonprofit institutions with a commitment to their communities and value-based care.[20] Also, because of the new payer mix under the ACA, AMCs have a high proportion of Medicare and Medicaid patients who were eligible to be part of a value-based payment model. AMCs therefore stood to have considerable financial benefit through the MSSP programs if they were able to achieve shared savings under an ACO program.

Despite the early promise, many AMCs have struggled to achieve the shared savings expected from the APMs. For example, Dartmouth-Hitchcock, one of the first ACOs established and home to the researchers who developed the concept for the practice model, halted its ACO in 2016 after it was unable to reach cost-saving benchmarks linked to increased reimbursement.[21] AMCs' difficulties achieving financial savings under APMs are partially due to the complexity of cases that are not fully accounted for. Also, there is evidence of "adverse selection," with more low-acuity cases being directed away from AMCs by referring physicians because of their overall higher costs, whereas complex cases continue to be referred because of AMCs' ability to provide complex care.[20]

Value-based programs continue to expand outside of the initial focus on APMs under the ACA and have started to focus more on high-cost specialty care services. For example, in 2016, the initiation of the Comprehensive Care for Joint Replacement model bundled payment for each procedure into a single episode, including surgery and all associated care extending out 90 days from the index procedure. AMCs represent a large proportion of the institutions involved in the comprehensive joint replacement program. Two-year data suggest that the program has decreased discharges to postacute care facilities and reduced costs.[22]

COMPETING FOR REIMBURSEMENT AND MARKET SHARE

The opening of the federal insurance exchanges was intended to increase accessibility for patients and encourage competition among insurance providers. The average number of insurance companies offered on the exchanges expanded between 2014 and 2016. After several insurance providers were unable to meet performance expectations and experienced financial losses, they chose to exit the exchanges and focus on more profitable sectors, such as employer-based insurance.[23] This resulted in a contraction in the number of participating insurers from an average of 5 to 3.5 providers per state between 2014 and 2018, with 8 states currently having only a single carrier.[24] This consolidation of insurance providers gave insurance companies greater leverage over health care providers. Controlling a greater market share allows insurers to bargain for lower reimbursement rates and use provider network limitations to restrict or exclude high-cost providers. For example, in 2014, Anthem–Blue Cross Blue Shield, the only New Hampshire insurance provider participating in the exchange, excluded 10 hospitals from its limited network. The company cited other health care providers' willingness to accept reduced reimbursement rates and the companies' ability to reduce costs by limiting its network as justification for excluding 10 of the 26 critical access hospitals in the area.[25]

Influenced by the increased purchasing power of insurers, health care providers have responded through consolidation of their own. Between 2008 and 2015, hospital consolidation increased by more than 100%.[26] Many of these consolidations are linked to an academic health system because their large size, reputation, and financial stability give them a strong position when dealing with insurance providers and attracting patients. For example, the University of Pittsburgh Medical Center–Pinnacle has expanded to 32 hospitals throughout the Pittsburgh area as of 2018 and continues to grow.[27] Between 2002 and 2015, hospitals with weaker financial performance were more likely to be acquired; however, more recently, acquisitions have been between strong partners rather than purchasing hospitals struggling with changes under the ACA.[25,28] This includes purchases or expansions outside of AMCs' home states and even internationally. For example, the Cleveland Clinic has a location in Abu Dhabi and plans to open a hospital in London in 2021.[29]

POLITICAL UNCERTAINTY AND LEGAL CHALLENGES INFLUENCING AMC PRACTICES

Since the election of the Trump Administration in 2016, there have been significant changes and challenges to the ACA. With the passage of the Tax Cuts and Jobs Act, the penalty under the individual mandate was removed. There has also been an expansion of Short Term–Limited Duration insurance plans that allows individuals to purchase very low-cost plans that do not cover the essential health benefits mandated under the ACA. There have also been initiatives to impose work hour requirements on Medicaid recipients, with pilots being run in select states. How these changes will influence AMCs is still to be realized, but it is suspected that these changes will result in fewer young individuals purchasing health insurance plans and may exclude some populations from Medicaid who are unable to work, but do not qualify for disability exemptions. These individuals are all populations that are more likely to receive care at an AMC and therefore may influence payer mix. In 2019, the federal health care exchanges saw their first decline in enrollment since their opening in 2014.

DISCLOSURE

The authors have nothing to disclose.

REFERENCES

1. Definitive Healthcare. The unique struggle of Academic Medical Centers. 2017. Available at: https://blog.definitivehc.com/academic-medical-center-struggle. Accessed October 9, 2019.
2. Medicaid.gov. Medicaid disproportionate share payments. 2019. Available at: https://www.medicaid.gov/medicaid/finance/dsh/index.html. Accessed October 9, 2019.
3. Wynn BO, Smalley R, Cordasco KM. Does it cost more to train residents or to replace them? A look at the costs and benefits of operating graduate medical education programs. Santa Monica (CA): RAND Corp; 2013. Available at: https://www.rand.org/pubs/research_reports/RR324.html.
4. Centers for Medicare & Medicaid Services. Medicare acute inpatient PPS. 2018. Available at: https://www.cms.gov/Medicare/Medicare-Fee-for-Service-Payment/AcuteInpatientPPS/. Accessed April 2, 2019.
5. Hoehn RS, Wima K, Vestal MA, et al. Effect of hospital safety-net burden on cost and outcomes after surgery. JAMA Surg 2016;151(2):120–8.
6. National Academy of Medicine. Accounting for social risk factors in Medicare payment: identifying social risk factors. Washington, DC: National Academies Press (US); 2016.
7. Bush H, Gerber LH, Stepanova M, et al. Impact of healthcare reform on the payer mix among young adult emergency department utilizers across the United States (2005-2015). Medicine (Baltimore) 2018;97(49):e13556.
8. American Academy of Pediatrics. Physician compensation models. 2019. Available at: https://www.aap.org/en-us/professional-resources/practice-transformation/managing-your-career/Pages/Physician-Compensation-Models.aspx. Accessed October 9, 2019.
9. The CommonWealth Fund. Fiscal case for medicaid expansion. 2019. Available at: https://www.commonwealthfund.org/blog/2019/fiscal-case-medicaid-expansion. Accessed October 9, 2019.
10. Rosenbaum S, Westmoreland TM. The Supreme Court's surprising decision on the Medicaid expansion: how will the federal government and states proceed? Health Aff (Millwood) 2012;31(8):1663–72.
11. Health Reform Monitoring Survey. Taking stock: health insurance coverage under the ACA as of March 2016. 2016. Available at: http://hrms.urban.org/briefs/health-insurance-coverage-ACA-March-2016.html. Accessed October 9, 2019.
12. Healthinsurance.org. Individual mandate. 2019. Available at: https://www.healthinsurance.org/glossary/individual-mandate/. Accessed October 9, 2019.
13. Healthcare.gov. The fee for not having insurnace. 2019. Available at: https://www.healthcare.gov/fees/fee-for-not-being-covered/. Accessed October 9, 2019.
14. The Kaiser Family. Health insurance coverage of the total population, foundation. 2019. Available at: https://www.kff.org/other/state-indicator/total-population/?currentTimeframe=0&sortModel=%7B%22colId%22:%22Location%22,%22sort%22:%22asc%22%7D. Accessed October 9, 2019.
15. Probst BD, Walls L, Cirone M, et al. Examining the effect of the Affordable Care Act on two Illinois emergency departments. West J Emerg Med 2019;20(5):710–6.
16. Gil JA, Goodman AD, Kleiner J, et al. The affordable care act decreased the proportion of uninsured

patients in a safety net orthopaedic clinic. Clin Orthop Relat Res 2018;476(5):925–31.

17. Blavin F. Association between the 2014 Medicaid expansion and US hospital finances. JAMA 2016;316(14):1475–83.

18. Toussaint RJ, Bergeron SG, Weaver MJ, et al. The effect of the Massachusetts Healthcare Reform on the uninsured rate of the orthopaedic trauma population. J Bone Joint Surg Am 2014;96(16):e141.

19. Pande AH, Ross-degnan D, Zaslavsky AM, et al. Effects of healthcare reforms on coverage, access, and disparities: quasi-experimental analysis of evidence from Massachusetts. Am J Prev Med 2011;41(1):1–8.

20. New England Journal of Medicine–Catalyst. What value-based payment means for academic medical centers. 2019. Available at: https://catalyst.nejm.org/value-based-payment-academic-medical-centers/. Accessed October 5, 2019.

21. Dropout by Dartmouth raises questions on health law cost-savings effort. The New York Times 2016. Available at: https://www.nytimes.com/2016/09/11/us/politics/dropout-by-dartmouth-raises-questions-on-health-law-cost-savings-effort.html. Accessed October 9, 2019.

22. Finkelstein A, Ji Y, Mahoney N, et al. Mandatory Medicare bundled payment program for lower extremity joint replacement and discharge to institutional postacute care: interim analysis of the first year of a 5-year randomized trial. JAMA 2018;320(9):892 900.

23. The Kaiser Family Foundation. Insurer financial performance in the early years of the Affordable Care Act. 2017. Available at: https://www.kff.org/health-reform/issue-brief/insurer-financial-performance-in-the-early-years-of-the-affordable-care-act/. Accessed October 9, 2019.

24. The Kaiser Family Foundation. Insurer participation on the ACA marketplaces. 2018. Available at: https://www.kff.org/health-reform/issue-brief/insurer-participation-on-aca-marketplaces-2014-2019/. Accessed October 9, 2019.

25. Concord Monitor. Anthem takes heat from N.H. senators over limited provider network for marketplace plans. 2013. Available at: https://www.concordmonitor.com/Archive/2013/09/AnthemSenate-CM-091913. Accessed October 9, 2019.

26. Kaufman, Hall & Associates, LLC. 2018 M&A in review: a new healthcare landscape takes shape. 2019. Available at: https://www.kaufmanhall.com/sites/default/files/documents/2019-01/2018-merger-acquisition-year-in-review_kaufman-hall.pdf. Accessed October 9, 2019.

27. University of Pittsburg Medical Center. UMPC selects architecture firm for $2B specialty hospital investment. 2018. Available at: https://www.upmc.com/media/news/092618-hospital-building-projects. Accessed October 9, 2018.

28. Noles MJ, Reiter KL, Boortz-marx J, et al. Rural hospital mergers and acquisitions: which hospitals are being acquired and how are they performing afterward? J Healthc Manag 2015;60(6):395–407.

29. Cleveland Clinic London. Our integrated healthcare delivery system. 2019. Available at: https://clevelandcliniclondon.uk/about. Accessed October 9, 2019.

How a Nationalized Health Care System Influences Hand Surgery Practice
The United Kingdom Perspective

Daniel Cadoux- Hudson, MRCS(Eng), MBBS, BSc,
David Warwick, MD, FRCS(Orth)*

KEYWORDS

- National health service • Hand surgery • United Kingdom • Nationalized system

KEY POINTS

- The National Health Service is the provider of nationalized health care across the United Kingdom. It is entirely funded through general taxation.
- Hand surgery is delivered by both plastic and trauma and orthopaedic surgeons in a variety of different settings, including regional specialist centers.
- The process of commissioning these services is complex and heavily influenced by a restriction in resources.
- The nationalized nature of this system allows research, standardization of provision, and monitoring of devices.

INTRODUCTION

Various health care systems provide hand surgery services around the world, varying from a comprehensive insurance system, a partly insured system or personal funding, through to a social health insurance system that is funded entirely by the taxpayer. In the United Kingdom, hand surgery is predominantly provided by the state with funding derived from general taxation: the National Health Service (NHS). This service is supplemented by entirely optional private insurance or personal funding. There is a growing partnership, with the NHS purchasing capacity from the private sector.

This article discusses the history and evolution of the nationalized health care system in the United Kingdom, and the subsequent political, economic, and social factors that influence it.

Hand surgery is a small area of practice within the NHS. The authors provide their personal perspective on the influence of the nationalized system on this specialty.

THE NATIONAL HEALTH SERVICE

Nationalized health care in the United Kingdom is delivered through the NHS This service is publicly owned and is funded through general taxation. There are 4 separate entities to the NHS because administration is devolved to the governments of the separate nations of the United Kingdom. These entities are:

- NHS England
- NHS Scotland
- NHS Wales
- Health and Social Care Northern Ireland

These organizations all share the same fundamental tenet: they are free at the point of delivery (with the exception of prescription charges and dental services).

Hand Unit, University Hospital Southampton, Tremona Road, Southampton SO166YD, UK
* Corresponding author.
E-mail address: davidwarwick@handsurgery.co.uk

Hand Clin 36 (2020) 171–180
https://doi.org/10.1016/j.hcl.2020.01.004
0749-0712/20/Crown Copyright © 2020 Published by Elsevier Inc. All rights reserved.

History and Founding Principles

To appreciate the influences on the provision of nationalized health care in the United Kingdom, it is necessary to understand its history. Before the NHS, health care in the United Kingdom was delivered through a combination of charity, philanthropy, social insurance schemes, and private practice. There had been little in the way of centralized planning of health care and many patients were left with large, unaffordable health care bills. Throughout the early part of the twentieth century, as treatments became increasingly expensive and complicated, there was a desire among the political classes to change the way in which health care was funded, particularly after the First World War. The introduction of National Insurance in 1911 (a charge levied on the wages of all workers) initially included cover for some access to medical care.

Following the Second World War, when the burden of health care was increasing at the same time as the United Kingdom was suffering from the economic effects of 6 years of war, there was a push from the Labour government of the time to act on the Beveridge Report of 1942. The report described a "national health service organised under the health departments." This was the basis on which the NHS was founded on 5 July 1948 by Aneurin Bevan, the Health Secretary at the time following the National Health Service Act of 1946. At the same time, the health services of Scotland and Northern Ireland were formed. Initially Wales and England had the same health service, although these were divided in 1969 into separate services, with the Welsh service fully devolved to the Welsh government in 1999.

Modern Structure of the National Health Service

Although the organization of the NHS is devolved to the 4 nations, the funding is all provided by the UK central government. The NHS budget was £158.7 billion in 2018 to 2019. **Fig. 1** shows the NHS structure.

National Health Service in England
The greatest proportion of this budget (£130.9 billion)[1] was spent in England, which has the largest population (56.0 million).[2] The most recent significant reform of the NHS in England was in 2012 with the introduction of the Health and Social Care Act. This act fundamentally changed the structure of the NHS in England. The NHS is the political responsibility of the Secretary of State for Health and Social Care. It is primarily divided into:

- NHS England (NHSE)
- Health Education England (HEE)
- Public Health England (PHE)

NHS England is directly responsible for running primary care services such as general practice. Around 60% of NHS England's budget is given to clinical commissioning groups (CCGs), of which there are 211, who are responsible for commissioning both emergency and planned care. Services can be commissioned from both public and private providers, provided they meet the required standard. Specialist services are also commissioned directly by NHS England, including very complex hand surgery for which regional rather than local services are required.

Public Health England provides advice and support to the NHS and local authorities with regard to public health and epidemiology.

Health Education England supports the delivery of training and improvement for all health care workers, which consumes around £4.2 billion. There are several independent regulators and professional bodies, whose roles are discussed later in the article.[3]

National Health Service in Scotland
Funding for the NHS in Scotland ultimately comes from the UK general taxation but is devolved to the Scottish government through an arrangement called the Barnett formula.[4] The total budget is around £13.5 billion.[5] Scotland comprises 14 geographic and 7 nongeographic health boards, which are responsible for organizing and delivering health care. These boards own and run hospitals in Scotland.[6] Other bodies within NHS Scotland include NHS Health Scotland, the role of which is similar to Public Health England, and NHS Education Scotland, which is responsible for training and education. This system does not have the complex, expensive, and controversial arrangement of commissioning that is present in the English System.

National Health Service in Wales
The budget of NHS Wales is £8.3 billion,[7] and is the responsibility of the Welsh Government. Seven local health boards are responsible for the delivery of health care within a geographic area.[8] Again, there are several separate bodies within NHS Wales, including Public Health Wales and Health Education and Improvement Wales, which have similar roles to their counterparts in England and Scotland.

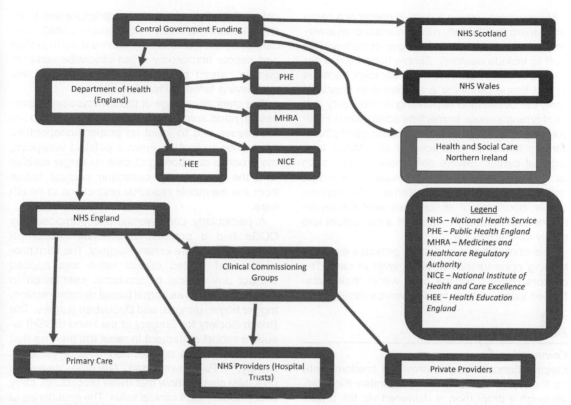

Fig. 1. Structure of NHS in the United Kingdom.

National Health Service in Northern Ireland

The overall annual budget is £6.0 billion.[9] Health care in Northern Ireland is the responsibility of the Northern Ireland Executive (the devolved government of Northern Ireland). It is delivered by Health and Social Care in Northern Ireland, and is different from the rest of the United Kingdom (with the exception of Scotland) because it is responsible for the delivery of both health and social care. There are 6 health and social care trusts across the country, which are responsible for services within their areas.[10] The Northern Ireland Medical and Dental Training Agency is responsible for medical training.

HAND SURGERY IN THE UNITED KINGDOM
Provision Overview

Hand surgery in the United Kingdom is provided by 2 broad specialties, plastic surgery and orthopaedics, with specialized hand surgery available in larger centers.

Funding

It is a fundamental tenet of the NHS that treatment is provided free at the point of delivery, which provides equitable access to a full range of treatment regardless of social status or personal resource.

Hand trauma is well covered by the public sector and is not restricted by cost. It is fully funded and provided free at the point of delivery.

In the public sector, both emergency and elective services are funded centrally in Wales, Scotland, and Northern Ireland, and by 211 local CCGs in England. The CCGs are administrative bodies with medically qualified direction that use centrally provided funds to purchase care locally. Some people opt to use private insurance (provided as an optional but taxable benefit by an employer). Others choose to purchase their own private insurance or simply to pay as they go, from their own income or savings. There are currently no personal tax incentives for private care despite this removing burden from the state.

Hand Trauma

Urgent hand surgery is usually performed by general plastic and orthopaedic surgeons with referral to more specialized services depending on the level of expertise required and the local arrangements regarding care.

Most patients attend a walk-in center or a casualty department (usually run by nurses) or an emergency department (with a larger compliment of staff to include doctors). Simple hand injuries are treated in these facilities; more complex fractures or soft tissue problems are referred to specialist care, the destination depending on the injury and local arrangements. Immediate admission is available when needed to an orthopaedic, plastic hand surgery facility in that hospital or transfer to a regional center. Severe soft tissue injuries such as flexor tendon division, neurovascular damage, and amputation are usually referred to the regional center, because not all hospitals have the expertise or staff numbers to support a competent and timely on-call service.

This comprehensive system provides excellent training opportunities at each level of care. The doctors provide trauma care within their state-funded salary with no fee-for-service facility.

Elective Hand Surgery

Commissioning

Elective hand surgery is provided predominantly by the public sector within the United Kingdom, although a proportion is delivered via the private sector. In the public sector in England, services are purchased by the CCGs from a variety of providers: large teaching hospitals, smaller district hospitals, privately run independent treatment centers (which are small surgical facilities providing care for simple procedures on low-risk patients), and on a case-by-case basis in private hospitals. A small proportion are undertaken in outpatient clinic facilities in general practice.

About 9% of hand surgery is provided separately from the NHS in private practice with patients choosing their surgeon and hospital, using their private insurance or personal funds.

The CCGs are empowered by the 2012 Health and Social Care Act to stop commissioning a particular procedure, to set the amount that they pay for that particular procedure, and to set conditions for each procedure. This approach allows some oversight of practice that, although perhaps perceived (unreasonably) as a threat by some hand surgeons to their autonomous individual practice, is (properly) intentioned to ration expense in a resource-limited public health care setting based on clinical evidence or consensus rather than on idiosyncratic surgeon opinion or bias. Thus trigger finger surgery cannot be performed unless there has been at least 1 steroid injection; carpal tunnel surgery cannot be performed unless there has been a trial of splinting or a steroid injection; Dupuytren surgery cannot be performed

unless there is a substantial contracture and functional deficit; *Clostridium histolyticum* collagenase cannot be used unless 1 injection is likely to suffice and needle fasciotomy is not otherwise suitable; ganglia cannot be excised unless symptomatic and having failed at least 1 aspiration.

The clear advantage of the commissioning process in hand surgery is to limit spending to proven techniques and to insist on proper nonoperative care when indicated. From a political viewpoint, the process of rationing of care no longer resides with the government, deflecting political fallout from the inevitable resource restrictions in health care.

A particularly controversial policy imposed by CCGs had a potential detrimental impact on proper patient care in hand surgery. The term procedures of limited clinical value was applied without any clinical or academic justification to procedures such as carpal tunnel decompression, trigger finger, ganglia, and Dupuytren surgery. The British Society for Surgery of the Hand (BSSH) issued a robust statement to rebut the premise that these procedures are not beneficial or value for money.[11] Patient-reported outcome measures (PROMs) clearly show that these procedures carry exceptionally high clinical value. The experience of this clumsy attempt to ration common procedures emphasizes the need for good-quality research and data into the practice of hand surgery in the United Kingdom.

Another disadvantage of the commissioning process is that the mass diversion of simple hand surgery cases to independent treatment centers or private hospitals that can provide at lower cost deprives the NHS teaching hospitals of training material, funds, and personnel to support other activities (especially training, hand trauma care, and complex hand surgery).

More recently, CCGs have insisted that some procedures can only be performed in an office environment (rather than a formal operating theater): carpal tunnel decompression, trigger finger release, needle fasciotomy, de Quervain. These procedures can be delivered with a clean environment and especially with wide-awake local anesthetic, no tourniquet (WALANT). There may be some benefit in cost and efficiency of turnover. However, some of the cost savings (because the CCGs pay a lower tariff to the provider) may be illusory because the total overheads in the whole system (real estate, staff costs, heating and lighting, management and so forth) remain unchanged but the taxpayer at central level is underwriting the extra cost of the commissioning process and the extra operating facility. Removal of these cases from larger centers also deprives those centers of some of the resources (staff, funding, patient material) they require to run training programs, deliver trauma, and perform more complex hand surgery.

Centralization of services: the hub and spoke model

Nationalized health care can potentially enhance the care and cost of some specific rare, complex, or expensive hand surgery procedures. This enhancement can be achieved by a process known as specialized commissioning, which is funded directly from central funds rather than from the CCG; for example, radiocarpal wrist replacement, total distal radioulnar joint replacement, and complex scaphoid reconstruction.[12] This arrangement reduces the financial burden that funding such treatments might place on individual CCGs and reduces the geographic variation of these services. It should have the advantage of concentrating the clinical experience and cost into a few specialist hand surgery centers, thereby driving the sensible centralization of services in a hub and spoke model.[12]

The central government also promotes the Getting It Right First Time (GIRFT) initiative, which will drive change in the way that certain aspects of hand surgery are delivered.[13] GIRFT is a project funded by NHS England that strives to ensure a degree of consistency across the NHS by assessing each hospital and then recommending changes. These changes include insisting that each hospital carries a smaller choice of implants for any particular procedure (to avoid the cost of surgeons each demanding their own favorites) and mandating that more complex services should be referred to a smaller number of more specialist centers, which will develop better and less morbid outcomes, at lower cost. In hand surgery, this model could apply to complex expensive procedures such as wrist replacement, distal radioulnar joint replacement, flexor tendon repair, and brachial plexus surgery.

There are potential disadvantages to the hub and spoke model; for example, reduced capacity in the specialist centers for providing basic hand surgery elective and trauma services that provide funding and training material. Nevertheless, the benefit to the patients and the taxpayers is self-evident. This model is evolving, driven by factors such as informal and formal interhospital arrangements, personal contacts, GIRFT, litigation risk, and commissioning. **Fig. 2** shows the hub and spoke model used in the NHS.

Waiting lists

The NHS mandates maximum waiting times for hand surgery. The current target, which the system

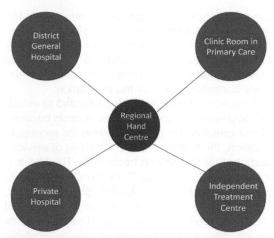

Fig. 2. Hub and spoke model for the delivery of hand surgery services.

is struggling to deliver, is 18 weeks.[14] For patients, this target has the advantage that, regardless of personal circumstance or resource, the treatment will happen by a predictable time. For surgeons, there is a lever to persuade hospital management (who are under heavy pressure from central government to deliver) to provide adequate resources to expand the service. However, there are some disadvantages. A system that is tuned to deliver a certain waiting time may be driven to prioritize patients who have been waiting a long time for trivial conditions (perhaps Dupuytren contracture) instead of clinically or socially urgent cases (debilitating conditions preventing work or requiring domestic care).

Modest (not too long, not too short) waiting times for routine problems can potentially save money for the nationalized system. The absence of precipitous surgery can expose the natural history of many conditions that, if left alone, either resolve by themselves (eg, most painful joints, posttraumatic ulnar corner pain, epicondylalgia) or that may respond to other modalities, such as steroid injections or physiotherapy. A proportion of the population and employers are motivated to purchase private insurance or self-pay for health care in order to avoid a wait, thus subtracting themselves from the taxpayer's burden, which shortens overall waiting times and reduces overall NHS cost.

HAND SURGERY RESEARCH IN THE NATIONAL HEALTH SERVICE
Advantages of a Nationalized Research System

A nationalized system has significant advantages for research and this benefit has materialized in hand surgery. Because the NHS is provided to the entire UK population, there is a large cohort of patients available for research, most of whom may feel the goodwill to contribute to research that benefits a state-funded system. Data are held relatively consistently across the population.

A publicly funded system is motivated to establish cost-effective and reliable treatments because of the pressure for providing value for money. In addition, the system of commissioning of services adds further scrutiny on treatments. The National Institute of Health and Care Excellence (NICE) which is a publicly funded, although independent, section of the Department of Health and Social Care, provides guidance on the best treatments for conditions based on the evidence available and its relative cost. Examples of NICE guidance include radiotherapy and collagenase clostridium histolyticum for Dupuytren disease[15] and total wrist replacement for arthritis.[16]

To support research across the NHS, there is a state-funded Clinical Research Network. Larger hospitals are primed with salaried research nurses and administrators. Thus, each hospital can promptly recruit into large multicenter studies as soon as the opportunity to engage in that project arrives.

Hand surgeons are motivated by the state to engage in research. NHS consultant job contracts include the option for research; this work is recognized in hand surgeons' remuneration packages, in the Clinical Excellence Award system, and contributes to those seeking academic promotion. In addition, the BSSH has an active Research Committee that provides support for pump priming and other research.

National Hand Surgery Trials

Examples of trials relevant to hand surgery funded by the NHS with recruitment from across NHS hospitals include the Distal Radius Fracture Fixation Trial (DRAFFT) (**Box 1**),[17] Scaphoid Waist Internal Fixation for Fractures Trial (SWIFFT) (**Box 2**),[18] and Dupuytren Interventions Surgery Versus Collagenase (DISC) (**Box 3**).[19] These trials are large enough to provide answers to essential issues of efficacy, cost, and safety.

National Funding of Research

Hand surgery studies may be funded by the National Institute for Health Research (NIHR) or by other public or commercial sources. The research described in the boxes earlier was largely funded by the NIHR, which is an independent public body funded by the Department of Health and Social Care, although it does receive funding from the United Kingdom Foreign Aid budget to research

---

> **Box 1**
> **Distal radius fracture fixation trial**
>
> - Multi center randomized controlled trial
> - Published 2014
> - 461 patients
> - Distal radius fracture fixation: Kirschner wire versus distal radius locking plate fixation
> - Exclusion criteria: not needing fixation, beyond 3 cm of the wrist, intra-articular fracture
> - Summary: no statistical difference in outcome (patient-rated wrist evaluation) at 12 months

---

health care in low-income to middle-income countries.[20]

The Health Technology Assessment Programme is funded by the NIHR. Its aim is to assess new treatments for a condition as to whether they may benefit NHS patients, comparing them with the existing standard treatments to assess their effectiveness. The results of these studies are freely available on the NIHR Web site. The research performed in the NHS has impact beyond the United Kingdom and its health system.

Patient-reported Outcome Measures

The conflict between inexorable demand for treatment and the cost-conscious environment of the NHS mandates evidence for the efficacy and cost-effectiveness of interventions. This requirement is against a background of focusing on outcomes relevant to patients rather than doctors. Thus PROMs are essential in a nationalized system that, rightly, takes account of effectiveness from the patient's perspective. The NHS routinely collects PROMs on certain procedures (eg,

---

> **Box 2**
> **Scaphoid waist internal fixation for fractures trial**
>
> - Multicenter randomized controlled trial
> - Scaphoid waist fracture on plain film: cast versus early fixation
> - Final results not published (awaiting 5-year follow-up)
> - 438 patients
> - Plaster cast treatment versus early surgical fixation
> - Initial results after 1-year follow-up show no significant difference in outcomes

---

Box 3
Dupuytren interventions surgery versus collagenase

- Multicenter randomized controlled trial
- In progress
- Surgical removal of Dupuytren versus collagenase injection in patients with moderate disease
- In progress

---

herniae and varicosed veins), although not hand surgery as yet. Thus, in all of the 3 studies mentioned earlier, PROMs are key outcomes. Inappropriate perspectives of procedures (eg, the pejorative term procedures of limited clinical value) can be countered by routine PROMs collection. Accordingly, the BSSH has established the UK National Hand Registry using PROMs as its primary reporting measure. The aim of the registry is to measure all hand operations registered in order to allow assessment of individual procedures, units, and individual surgeons with regard to their outcomes in terms of both PROMs and complications.[21]

REGULATION OF MEDICAL DEVICES
Joint Registries

Hand surgeons are presented with a plethora of implants and gadgets, many, if not most, of which have no evidence. Countless devices in orthopaedics have been ignominiously withdrawn, sometimes under the cloud of litigation, when the lack of effectiveness, premature failure, or outright harm become apparent. In the United Kingdom, the National Joint Registry (NJR) requires mandatory data collection for all hip and knee implants; the outputs are compelling (especially when linked to GIRFT). Hand surgery implants are not yet under the remit of the NJR but it is hoped that this will happen. Meanwhile, the BSSH Hand Registry will provide national-level data on many of the implants that are used.

Central Monitoring

The Medicines and Healthcare Regulatory Agency (MHRA) plays an important role in regulating and monitoring medicines and medical devices in the United Kingdom. Much like NICE, the MHRA is an independent body that receives funding from the Department of Health and Social Care. By looking at evidence from the literature, various surgical registries, and the Yellow Card direct reporting mechanism it runs, the MHRA issues warnings

and recommendations on medical devices. It has previously issued advice regarding metal-on-metal bearing total hip replacements causing early failure in April 2010, recommending stopping implanting them.[22] Within hand surgery it monitors the use of all surgical devices, although it has not issued any formal warnings. Its position within the United Kingdom's publicly funded health system gives it a unique perspective to monitor these devices if problems occur.

Local Controls

NHS hospitals should require their surgeons to apply for permission to use a new implant or treatment. This requirement protects patients from cavalier innovation, protects hospitals from the cost of unproven technology or the even greater cost of treating failure, and the surgeons from reputation damage and litigation.

HUMAN RESOURCE MANAGEMENT
Consultant Contract

The contracts under which consultants (senior clinicians who have completed their training) work within the NHS are centrally negotiated. The salary is the same regardless of specialty and region (except for a London enhancement). Consultants' working time is divided into programmed activities (PAs). These activities are typically 4 hours in duration and can either be a direct clinical care (DCC) session or a supporting professional activity (SPA). DCCs include clinical sessions such as operating time and outpatients in addition to administrative time that may be needed to perform patient care. SPAs are dedicated time for other nonclinical activities, which may include time for professional administration and continuing professional development. SPAs are also used for teaching, research, and clinical audit purposes. With regard to hand surgery, this allows these activities to be performed in NHS time with the appropriate support. Most consultant contracts are 10 PAs per week, of which 1.5 to 2 are SPAs.[23]

The centrally negotiated contract has the advantage of providing consistent care for hand conditions across the country regardless of complexity, although to individual surgeons this may be seen as unfair if they manage complex cases or have a more intense daily workload or out-of-hours call rota. There is some room for individual incentivization within the NHS contract. The only mechanism that does exist for rewarding individual clinicians is the awarding of clinical excellence awards, which are awarded on a national or local basis either as an annual lump sum in the case of local awards and as an increase in salary in national awards. Current pension tax rules dilute the financial appeal of these awards. These awards are awarded for[24]:

- Commitment to patient care
- High standards of clinical and technical skills
- Sustained commitment to the values and goals of the NHS
- Contributions to service improvement
- Contributions to research
- Excellence in teaching, training, or management
- Contributions to leadership

Basic Training

Doctors in training in the United Kingdom are known as junior doctors. This term encompasses all doctors between qualifying from medical school through to when they complete their training program with the awarding of a Certificate of Completion of Training. Training of all junior doctors in England is provided by the NHS and run by Health Education England (HEE) with oversight from the General Medical Council (GMC). It is split between the training programs of both plastic surgery and trauma and orthopaedics. The salary is the same whatever the specialty and is supplemented depending on call commitments. Working hours are limited by a European Working Time Directive to just 48 h/wk. As with all surgical

specialties, this drastically limits the elective and trauma hand surgery procedures to which trainees are exposed.

A nationally controlled system has the advantage of consistency and high standards, exposing the trainees to a wide variety of individual orthopaedic, plastic, and hand surgery units with a variety of practices ranging from simple regular hand surgery to subspecialty work in regional hub centers.

Training can suffer from commissioning because there is an increasing number of patients who are having surgery in the private sector commissioned by the NHS. In 2018, 7.3% of total NHS expenditure was spent in the private sector.[25] The reduction in training opportunities for trainees is sure to have a detrimental effect. Providing training within the private sector is a potential solution for this, and there are a few examples of private providers having arranged for reciprocal arrangements for trainees to attend, such as in the Severn Deanery (a training region in south west England) where hand surgery trainees were able to go to the private sector to perform carpal tunnel decompression. They are few and often are not included within the training programme.[26]

Training Interface Groups

Training interface groups (TIGs) are specific training groups for subspecialties that share

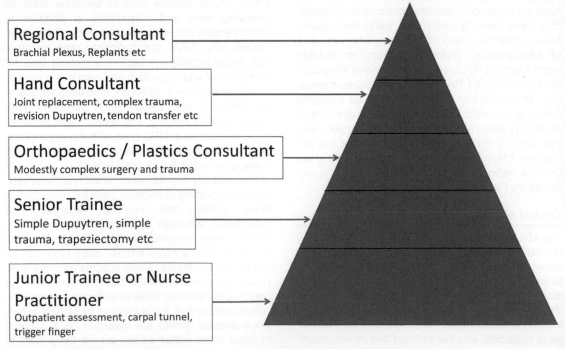

Regional Consultant
Brachial Plexus, Replants etc

Hand Consultant
Joint replacement, complex trauma, revision Dupuytren, tendon transfer etc

Orthopaedics / Plastics Consultant
Modestly complex surgery and trauma

Senior Trainee
Simple Dupuytren, simple trauma, trapeziectomy etc

Junior Trainee or Nurse Practitioner
Outpatient assessment, carpal tunnel, trigger finger

Fig. 3. Pyramid of hand surgery.

elements from more than 1 surgical specialty. There are currently TIGs in several aligned specialties that create fellowships, including hand surgery with both plastic and orthopaedic trainers. The TIG Fellows (who have basic training from either specialty) have an invaluable opportunity for higher-level training in hand surgery, all centrally funded and appointed.[27]

Fellowship Training

Following the award of the Certificate of Completion of Training, trainees often take further training in their subspecialties. In hand surgery, this can either be an international or a national fellowship. Typically, this is 1 to 2 years in duration. In the United Kingdom, there is the option of undertaking a diploma in hand surgery, which is provided and run by the BSSH. The diploma recognizes the subspecialist skills required for hand surgery. The training and supervision is provided by state-funded NHS consultants as part of their centrally negotiated job plan (SPAs).

The Pyramid of Hand Surgery Provision

In a state-funded, resource-restricted system, hand surgeons can develop a sensible system of delegation. More than other surgical specialty, hand surgery has a very large workload that comprises a broad range of procedures. The hub and spoke model, which can be readily constructed within a nationalized service, was described earlier. In addition, the level of expertise (and thus remuneration) can be adjusted to the complexity of a procedure. The senior author describes this as the pyramid of hand surgery. In the United Kingdom, there are examples of carpal tunnel decompression being undertaken by general practitioners and nurse practitioners. A great deal of simple trauma and simple surgery is performed by trainee doctors or generalist consultants. So long as there is appropriate training and governance, such a system can ensure cost-effective and safe care. **Figs. 2** and **3** show both the pyramid of hand surgery and the hub and spoke model.

SUMMARY

Health care in the United Kingdom is predominantly provided by a nationalized system. This nationalized system provides many advantages to patients: care free at the point of delivery, homogeneous standards across the nation, high standards of training, assurance of evidence-based and cost-effective care. It also provides advantages to hand surgeons: a set salary; a support system of secretaries and junior staff; the opportunity to develop a pyramidal system of hand surgery delivery in the hospital and hub-and spoke systems across a region; and clinical excellence awards to recognize extra contributions, such as research, teaching, and service development. Centrally managed training allows a standardized and high-quality experience onto which can be added the BSSH diploma. The NHS offers an unrivalled opportunity for large-scale hand surgery trials.

There are some disadvantages, including the administrative burden of managing commissioning and waiting lists, the loss of training and revenue opportunities as work is commissioned into alternative high-volume providers, and a lack of incentive for doing more complex procedures or providing more emergency care.

DISCLOSURE

The authors have nothing to disclose.

REFERENCES

1. Care DoHaS. Department of health and social care; annual reports and accounts 2018-2019. London: House of Commons; 2019.
2. Statistics OfN. Population estimates for the UK, England and Wales, Scotland and Northern Ireland: mid. 2018. Available at: https://www.ons.gov.uk/peoplepopulationandcommunity/populationandmigration/populationestimates/bulletins/annualmidyearpopulationestimates/mid2018. Accessed September 23, 2019.
3. Powell T. The structure of the NHS in England. London: House of Commons Library: House of Commons; 2017.
4. Facts about NHS funding in Scotland. Office of the Secretary of State for Scotland, GOV.UK website; 2014. Available at: https://www.gov.uk/government/news/facts-about-nhs-funding-in-scotland. Accessed September 23, 2019.
5. Scotland A. NHS in Scotland 2018. Report published by Audit Scotland,, Edinburgh, UK.
6. Structure of NHS Scotland. NHS Scotland; 2018. Available at: https://www.scot.nhs.uk/about-nhs-scotland/. Accessed September 23, 2019.
7. Annual budget motion 2019-20. Cardiff (UK): Welsh Assembly; 2019. Available at: https://gov.wales/sites/default/files/publications/2018-12/final-budget-2019-2020-motion.pdf. Accessed September 23, 2019.
8. Structure of the NHS in Wales. NHS Wales; 2019. Available at: http://www.wales.nhs.uk/nhswalesaboutus/structure. Accessed September 23, 2019.

9. Northern Ireland budget - Tables 2019-2020. Northern Ireland Department of Finance; 2019. Available at: https://www.finance-ni.gov.uk/publications/northern-ireland-budget-2019-20. Accessed September 23, 2019.

10. HSC structure. Health and Social Care Northern Ireland; 2019. Available at: http://online.hscni.net/home/hsc-structure/. Accessed September 23, 2019.

11. Shewring D, Hobby J, Warwick D, et al. NHS plan to restrict funding is not based on high quality data. BMJ 2018;362:k3743.

12. England N. Manual for prescribed specialised services 2018/19. 2017. Available at: https://www.england.nhs.uk/publication/manual-for-prescribed-specialised-services/. Accessed September 21, 2019.

13. Getting it right first. Time information leaflet. Published by Getting it Right First Time. Available at: https://gettingitrightfirsttime.co.uk/what-we-do/. Accessed September 21, 2019.

14. Guide to NHS waiting times in England. NHS England; 2016. Available at: https://www.nhs.uk/using-the-nhs/nhs-services/hospitals/guide-to-nhs-waiting-times-in-england/. Accessed September 22, 2019.

15. Radiation Therapy for early Dupuytren's disease: interventional procedures guidance. National Institute for Health and Clinical Excellence; 2016. Available at: https://www.nice.org.uk/guidance/ipg573/resources/radiation-therapy-for-early-dupuytrens-disease-pdf-1899872106511813. Accessed September 23, 2019.

16. Total wrist replacement: interventional procedures guidance. National Institute for Health and Care Excellence; 2008. Available at: https://www.nice.org.uk/guidance/ipg271/resources/total-wrist-replacement-pdf-1899865572805573. Accessed September 23, 2018.

17. Costa ML, Achten J, Plant C, et al. UK DRAFFT: a randomised controlled trial of percutaneous fixation with Kirschner wires versus volar locking-plate fixation in the treatment of adult patients with a dorsally displaced fracture of the distal radius. Health Technol Assess 2015;19(17):1–124. v-vi.

18. Dias J, Brealey S, Choudhary S, et al. Scaphoid Waist Internal Fixation for Fractures Trial (SWIFFT) protocol: a pragmatic multi-centre randomised controlled trial of cast treatment versus surgical fixation for the treatment of bi-cortical, minimally displaced fractures of the scaphoid waist in adults. BMC Musculoskelet Disord 2016;17:248.

19. DISC: Dupuytren's Interventions Surgery vs. Collagenase. A pragmatic multi-centre randomised controlled non-inferiority, cost effectiveness trial comparing injections of collagenase into the cord to surgical correction in the treatment of moderate Dupuytren's contracture in adult patients. NIHR; 2016. Available at: https://www.journalslibrary.nihr.ac.uk/programmes/hta/1510204/#/. Accessed August 19, 2019.

20. Our mission and strategic workstreams. National Institute of Health Research; 2019. Available at: https://www.nihr.ac.uk/about-us/our-mission/our-mission-and-strategic-workstreams.htm. Accessed September 23, 2019.

21. The UK national hand Registry (formerly the audit Database). British Society for Surgery of the Hand; 2017. Available at: https://www.bssh.ac.uk/about/news/114/uk_national_hand_registry_formerly_the_audit_database. Accessed September 23, 2019.

22. Medical device alert: all metal on metal hip replacements. Medicines and healthcare regulatory authority. Accessed September 23, 2019.

23. Consultant job planning: a best practice guide. NHS Improvement; 2017. Available at: https://improvement.nhs.uk/documents/1964/Job_planning_-_revised.pdf. Accessed September 23, 2019.

24. Consultant award schemes. The British Medical Association; 2019. Available at: https://www.bma.org.uk/advice/employment/pay/cea-clinical-excellence-awards. Accessed September 23, 2019.

25. Department of Health and Social Care. Annual reports and accounts 2018-2019. London: Department of Health and Social Care; 2019. Available at: https://assets.publishing.service.gov.uk/government/uploads/system/uploads/attachment_data/file/832765/dhsc-annual-report-and-accounts-2018-to-2019.pdf. Accessed September 22, 2019.

26. Royal College of Surgeons. Position statement 2018. Position Statement - Royal College of Surgeons: Published 2018, London. Available at: https://www.rcseng.ac.uk/-/media/files/rcs/about-rcs/government-relations-consultation/rcs-position-paper-on-training-in-the-independent-sector-november-2018-final.pdf. Accessed September 23, 2019, 2019.

27. Hand Surgery Training Interface Group. Joint Committee on Surgical Training. 2018. Available at: https://www.jcst.org/training-interface-groups/hand-surgery/. Accessed September 23, 2019.

Leveraging the Electronic Health Record System to Enhance Hand Surgery Practice

Gregory D. Byrd, MD, MA[a],*, David Wei, MD, MS[b]

KEYWORDS

- Efficiency • Productivity • Electronic health record • Electronic medical record

KEY POINTS

- Electronic health records (EHRs) have seen a dramatic increase in usage in clinics across the country since the implementation of the Health Information Technology for Economic and Clinical Health (HITECH) Act in 2009.
- Despite the initial frustration associated with integrating an EHR into your practice, there can be some benefits outlined in this article.
- There is a push so that future EHRs will be able to integrate better improving the portability of patient health care information.

INTRODUCTION

Electronic medical records (EMRs) and electronic health records (EHRs) are here to stay. In 2017, 86% of office-based physician practices had adopted some form of an EHR. This number is up from 21% in 2004.[1] One important thing to note is that from a pure nomenclature standpoint, EMRs and EHRs are not the same. An article by the Office of the National Coordinator for Health Information Technology (ONC) clarified the difference between EMRs and EHRs. EMRs came first and were largely digital versions of the paper charts in the clinician's office. EMRs normally focused on one's practice office and did not really leave that one practice.

EHRs do what EMRs do but are designed to focus on the whole health of the patient and communicate that across different platforms. They are designed to reach out beyond the health organization and share with other health care providers and organizations easily and electronically and do not require printing of the chart to transfer from one organization to another.[2] For the purposes of this article we use the term EHR.

EHRs were started in the 1960s and were initially only at major health systems because of the high cost of hardware and implementation and the required infrastructure. In the 1970s, the federal government started using an EHR in the Department of Veterans Affairs called VistA.

With the advent of the personal computer and a mouse, what were once keystrokes were transformed into clicks. The personal computer and the ever-improving computing power made the implementation of EHRs more feasible and cheaper from a hardware standpoint. It is still well documented that there is a significant cost from lost productivity and changed workflow during implementation.[3]

In 1997, the Institute of Medicine released a report advocating a shift from paper-based medical records to EMRs.[4] This was followed by the creation of the ONC of Health Information Technology.[5]

The major increase in adoption of EHRs occurred after the passing in 2009 of the Health Information Technology for Economic and Clinical Health (HITECH) Act. This act included a

[a] Olympia Orthopaedic Associates, Olympia, WA, USA; [b] Orthopaedic and Neurosurgery Specialists, 40 Valley Drive, Greenwich, CT 06830, USA
* Corresponding author. 7238 Huckleberry Road Northwest, Olympia, WA 98502.
E-mail address: gregory.byrd@gmail.com

Hand Clin 36 (2020) 181–188
https://doi.org/10.1016/j.hcl.2020.01.016

component focusing on electronic health records and meaningful use, and provided financial incentives for the adoption of EHRs (**Fig. 1**).

With the ever-increasing computing power and cloud-based systems in place, EHRs do much more than simply keep medical records. They now are the backbone of a practice. They are responsible for the clinic templates and patient scheduling. Billing and coding run through the systems with collections often integrated. This allows for a more seamless process for collections during check-in and monitoring patient balances. EHRs enable a level of running reports on many different aspects of a clinical practice that has never been possible before this level of practice integration and digitization. There are analytical programs that can help you manage your practice and increase the efficiency and understanding of how your practice is running. If you and your practice managers are not leveraging these resources, much of the benefits of an EHR are not being fully used by you and your practice.

Communication to referring providers is often automated in modern EHRs, so they will receive your most recent note when the chart is signed. This facilitates timelier sharing of treatment plans and provides patient updates to those practitioners who are entrusting their patients with your care. Lack of communication is a common complaint among referring providers and when this tool is used effectively can limit this complaint.

Most modern EHRs have some method of allowing patients easier access to their medical records through an online login. This feature allows patients to easily review their notes after their visits to review the treatment plan, remind them of things discussed in the visits they may have forgotten, and review their charts for accuracy. An online patient communication method is also part of many modern EHRs. This enables patients to bypass the phone system and reach the medical team with questions and concerns through online messages, which can have many benefits when

monitored properly. By direct communication in their chart, it can dramatically reduce the voicemail burden on staff, allowing them to more easily answer these questions during intermittent available times during the day. These messages can be accessed by supporting staff who can help with these questions, easing the burden on the staff who are in a busy clinic. The messages are a time-stamped document and thus provide accurate documentation regarding the time and nature of the requests. Some practices will only honor prescription refill requests through the online portal. It is important that monitoring these messages is viewed as critical in a practice to make sure no adverse events occur because a message was not seen in a timely fashion. Educating patients in terms of when to use the portal is critical as well. Simple questions and refills are very appropriate. Concerns for infection after surgery or an adverse event after an injection are probably better served with a phone call.

With this level of integration and reliance on EHRs, it is easy to understand why they are such a focal point of practice efficiency and provider satisfaction.

Being electronic creates a level of portability that paper charts never allowed. This is beneficial for reviewing patient records while at the hospital, home, or on the road. It also allows offsite registration and data gathering that can be scanned or uploaded and reviewed by the provider in a physically different location. In my practice, our registration and referral center is located in a separate location from my clinic. They will receive phone calls from patients or receive records from the local urgent cares and emergency departments and upload their outside medical records into the EHR. These can then be reviewed with my medical assistant and triage the patients for the type and urgency of treatment that they will likely need. This helps expedite care for the acute injuries and enables me to save operating time for those cases that will likely require surgery before they

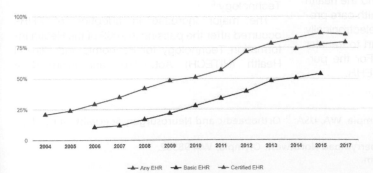

Fig. 1. Percentage of office-based physicians with electronic health record system 2004 to 2017. (*From* Office of the National Coordinator for Health Information Technology. 'Office-based Physician Electronic Health Record Adoption,' Health IT Quick-Stat #50. Available at: dashboard.healthit.gov/quickstats/pages/physician-ehr-adoption-trends.php. January 2019. Accessed Sept 29, 2019.)

are seen. Being able to predict what is coming into the clinic in the next couple of days and placing them appropriately is helpful. This would be far more cumbersome and require more on-site staff without an EHR.

INFORMATION RETRIEVAL

The purpose of a medical record is to document the history, examination, and plan for the patient's symptoms and diagnosis. EHRs accomplish this goal and when structured appropriately can excel. They create time stamps and a permanent record that will not be lost. The time stamps and ability to track modifications can be helpful for legal purposes. On a more daily functional basis, it is important to learn the fastest and easiest way to extract the necessary data out of the chart. Accessing a patient's record is much easier with an EHR because you can search by date of birth, name, and often other personal identifiers and have all their information available within seconds. There is the added benefit of cost savings on storage of charts for 5 to 10 years and the fees associated with accessing archived. However, the EHR and the associated notes are only as good as what goes in, and the format of the notes. I have structured my notes so that I know exactly where the pertinent information is and can easily scan their last note and be up to speed in a brief amount of time. When my medical assistant is rooming the patient, the assistant will also populate the reason for visit field with a couple of key words regarding the reason for the patient's visit and specifically how the patient is doing. If the patient is doing well and coming in for a follow-up appointment, I know it will likely be a quick visit and superficial chart scan is sufficient. If, on the other hand, the patient is having problems and not doing well, I will spend a little more time going through the chart to better understand what treatments have already been tried and what studies have been done. This also allows me to enter the room knowledgeable about previous treatments and having a future plan. By being clued in before entering the room, I can be more efficient in my chart review and not spend 5 minutes combing through the chart of a patient who is doing well and just wants to say thank you, which increases my efficiency while maximizing care.

In terms of chart review and setup before going in the room, I always have at least 2 windows open with the next 2 patients pulled up and their pertinent information. When I am in the room seeing a patient, my assistant will pull up the next patient's last chart note if I have seen the patient before. If they are new patients, their referral paperwork is opened and the assessment and plan is displayed. The imaging studies performed on the day of the visit or their most recent and pertinent images will also be prepared for viewing in a window. This allows me to walk out of the room and to the computer and start immediately preparing for the next patient without spending the additional time searching in the EHR for the pertinent portions of the patient's chart. One of the negative aspects of EHRs is the abundance of information documented that is not always relevant. This can increase the time required to extract the critical information needed for your visit with the patient. By using these tactics, you can decrease the amount of time required to prepare for the visit by leveraging the staff around you. If you can save 60 seconds per patient, which is conservative, in a busy clinic with 60 patients, that is an hour of saved time. This also speaks to having those around you function at their highest capacity. If somebody else can pull up the charts and films and free you up to see more patients, which is a revenue-generating event, then empower them to do that and improve the efficiency in your clinic.

COMMUNICATION

Most of the EMRs have consolidated many essential tasks of running a practice into one place. Prescriptions can now be electronically sent, including those that are controlled substances. This allows refills on controlled substances without the patient having to come pick up a physical prescription. This can be beneficial if you have a practice that extends over a large geographic area so that patients do not have to drive for an hour or more to pick up their prescriptions. With narcotic refills being easier to accommodate, this facilitates prescribing a smaller quantity for the initial prescription to try to decrease the amount of unused pain pills in patients' medicine cabinets. With the information all stored in the chart, it also keeps an accurate record of what has been prescribed in the practice and by whom. Having an EHR allows for greater access for staff and providers to see what has been prescribed and when considering refills, timing, or other alternatives for pain control than have already been prescribed.

The process of ordering procedures, studies, and therapy is also integrated into most EHRs. This sets up templates for near instant communication to the necessary parties needed to execute the order. Because everything is time stamped, it facilitates tracking and monitoring for this process. Templates can be beneficial in this process to increase efficiency and maintain accuracy. For surgery orders, this has dramatically reduced the last-minute calls regarding what implants or instruments are needed for the case. It has also increased my office efficiency because it was nearly impossible to have sheets of paper with all the potential things needed for the variety of upper extremity surgery that we perform. For total joints surgeons, they would have preprinted order sheets for total knees or hips. This is far more difficult to do for a comprehensive upper extremity practice. The ability to have an infinite number of templates for orders is a significant advantage for an EHR over preprinted order sheets. Although there is the initial upfront investment of time to create the templates, it will pay itself back many times over. Often a scribe or other staff can help with these tasks and the provider can edit and modify accordingly.

Ordering therapy also can be enhanced in an EMR. The prescriptions are faxed to the office you choose as soon as the order is signed. This process removes some of the barriers for patients to start therapy and ensures the office you choose is the one where they will be receiving their therapy. This prevents them from deciding to go to the physical therapist who does foot and ankle who their friend recommended because he or she is nice. They no longer have to initiate the appointment by calling or dropping off the prescription at the appropriate office. The designated office to which you sent the prescription will call because that office has their insurance information and can start to get the necessary authorization immediately.

Similarly, with ordering imaging studies and laboratory work, the process of ordering can be streamlined. Either the provider or their appropriately credentialed staff can enter the order, which is then sent to the facility or a scheduler to work on authorization and scheduling. As discussed with referrals, this can be accomplished at an off-site facility where overhead and rent are potentially lower. This also can be outsourced or leveraged with other practices to help lower overhead.

Interoffice communication also can be improved with EHRs. They all have the ability to leave notes on patients that are available for staff to view but not part of the official medical record. This can be beneficial for some of the more difficult patients to prepare providers before the patient encounter. Preferences for the patients also can be noted that can make for a better in-office experience without having it be part of the official medical record. Some systems also have Health Insurance Portability and Accountability Act–compliant texting features that can facilitate interoffice communication in real time. This can be helpful for urgent matters as they arise. Communicating to your medical assistant who is rooming your next patient that an injection is needed in your current room, or a cast or splint is needed and specifically what kind. In my practice this can all be done by my scribe while I am still talking with the patient and reviewing the treatment plan.

INBOX/BUCKET MANAGEMENT

Avoiding alarm fatigue and swelling inbox numbers that go ignored is a difficult thing to prevent with our current EHR systems. One of the blessings and curses of EHRs is the inbox or buckets. The messages and alerts seem to be never ending and keeping up with them is often exhausting in a busy practice. It is obviously always best to try to tackle and stay on top of the alerts as they come in; however, this is often not practical or realistic. This is another area in which your support staff can help to make sure that critical things are not missed. My medical assistant will scan my buckets and let me know if there are critical values or alerts that need my urgent attention. Some things can also get mislabeled and end up in the wrong bucket. This is where your staff can move or reassign these notifications in your bucket to make sure nothing is missed, and you are only spending time addressing what absolutely needs your attention. Another blessing and curse is the ability to easily review records and inboxes outside of the office. This can be helpful, but boundaries need to be set so that it does not become all-consuming and invasive into your down time. Many of the mundane tasks that fill our inboxes can be multitasked with other things and thus accomplished in the background of other activities (eg, watching TV).

INFORMATION ENTRY

EHRs allow for multiple methods of data entry into the patient chart. This can help to ease the burden of documentation on the provider and the provider's team. Many systems allow the patients to directly enter some of their health information before arrival. If you are using a platform that is shared with their other providers, then often much of their past medical history can be pulled in saving time on data entry. Another beneficial feature of some systems is the ability to search by key words for outside reports. Often when looking for nerve studies or therapy notes, you can search the patient's health record and these will be retrieved. This can save time from trying to search for the most recent records.

The medical assistant can then finish reviewing the information and add any additional pertinent information.

Documenting the patient encounter historically involved dictating the visit out of the room after the visit. With EMRs, some still practice this way; however, as technology has evolved, so have the methods of data entry. Voice recognition software has largely replaced the need for transcription services and is done in real time, saving the added delay associated with dictation services. This time savings can help to reduce the time bills are in accounts receivable, as well as the time between documentation and the note being ready. With after-visit summaries becoming more commonplace, these are difficult to generate with the traditional dictate and transcribe methods.

The provider sitting in front of a computer in the room during the visit is one method of entering information real time, but this can detract from the patient encounter. This form of data entry has demonstrated that the physician does not look at the patient as much, and if the computer monitor is kept away from the patient's view, it can lead to a sense of separation between the provider and the patient.[6-8] If you are in a situation in which you must document in the room on a computer, then templates and smart phrases will give you the best chance to document accurately while minimizing the detraction from the patient encounter. If you have to type it more than once in a month, it probably makes sense to make it into a template or smart phrase. For the most common diagnosis, often pretemplated notes can be created and the specific issues for the patient's presenting complaints and symptoms can be added. Although this diminishes the personal touches on a note, if done right can still accurately diagnose the visit and plan while still having a meaningful interaction with your patient.

Scribes have become a more recent answer to this age-old problem of chart note documentation. In the appropriate practice setting, this is arguably the one most impactful way to leverage your EMR to enhance your hand practice. There are a few studies that document the positive impact of scribes on clinical practices. If you ask anyone who has been involved in the transformation from paper charts to EMRs to life with a scribe, they will tell you they could not imagine ever going back. The studies help to support this emotion. Koshy and colleagues[9] found that using a scribe had a positive impact on clinician satisfaction and also less difficulty with the burden of documentation. In the review article by Holmstrom and colleagues, there were 3 studies cited that measured the effect of scribes on productivity. In

the studies evaluating a clinic setting, it was noted in all instances that productivity in terms of patients seen and RVUs generated went up.[6,10-12] In the only study reviewed looking at revenue generated, it was noted that with a scribe more revenue was generated for both direct and indirect services.[6,12] This should be expected, given RVUs and patients seen are increased with scribes. Last, the patient-clinician interaction was specifically evaluated in a study by Konrardy and colleagues[6,11] and noted to have a significantly higher quality of visit with a scribe versus without.

If you have the ability to see more patients from a demand standpoint, a scribe is beneficial from an efficiency and lifestyle standpoint, as well as being financially positive. There is still the burden of reviewing the notes, but this can often be accomplished at the end of the day or between patients.

Another option is a virtual scribe using a microphone that you wear in the room. This is often slightly less costly than hiring a scribe to have in your office. There is also the advantage of not having to worry if the scribe is sick or misses a day of work. However, there is often a delay of some sort from the time of visit until documentation and content of the note can be variable.

Part of the key to leveraging the EMR is not having overdocumentation that can become cumbersome to go through when reviewing patient records. There can be a significant discrepancy between what needs to be documented from a medical necessity, billing, and legal documentation standpoint and what is in the chart. From an efficiency point of view, veering on the side of less is more will prove to be far more efficient.

ELECTRONIC HEALTH RECORD AND THE QUALITY PAYMENT PROGRAM

The Centers for Medicare and Medicaid Services has implemented an incentive program known as the Quality Payment Program that attempts to reward value and outcomes of clinical practice through 2 systems, either Merit-based Incentive Payment Systems (MIPS) or Advanced Alternative Payments.[13] In this article, we focus on MIPS. If you are a MIPS-eligible physician, then your performance is measured through a report in 4 main areas: Quality, Improvement Activities, Promoting Interoperability, and Cost.

Quality is the category that was formerly named PQRS, and as a provider you would pick 6 measures of performance that fit your practice. *Promoting Interoperability* was formerly known as Meaningful Use, and focuses on patient engagement and electronic exchange of health information using a certified EHR technology. This category evaluates the proactive sharing of information with other clinicians or the patient in a comprehensive manner. For example, sharing test results, visit summaries, and therapeutic plans with the patient and other facilities to coordinate. *Improvement Activities* includes an assessment of care processes, enhancement of patient engagement in care, and increased access. Possible choices might include care coordination, patient and clinician shared decision making, and expansion of practice access. *Cost* is the final category, and replaces VBM (Value-Based Medicine). Medicare claims will be used to calculate the total cost of the care during the year or during a hospital stay.

Of these categories, the EHR has the most impact on Promoting Interoperability. This category alone can contribute 25% of your overall MIPS score. First, to fulfill this category, the EHR must be certified to the 2015 Edition certification criteria.[14] Then, clinicians must report on several required measures that are organized into 4 objectives: e-Prescribing, Provider to Patient Exchange, Health Information Exchange (HIE), and Public Health and Clinical Data Exchange. The following is a list of measures that may be applicable to a typical hand surgery practice.

For example, one required measure under the HIE objective, is the *Support Electronic Referral Loops by Sending Health Information*. This requires the clinician to create a summary of care record using the EHR and to electronically exchange it. Another required measure under the HIE objective is *Support Electronic Referral Loops by Receiving and Incorporating Health Information*. Under Provider to Patient exchange objective, the measure, *Provide Patients Electronic Access to Their Health Information,* specifies the patient must have timely (4 business days) access to view online, download, and transmit his or her health information. This health information may be accessible using any application that is configured to meet the technical specifications of the Application Programming Interface (API) of the EHR. *Electronic-prescribing*, or e-prescribing, is another measure that is required. This requires that prescriptions written by the clinician are queried for a drug formulary and then transmitted electronically by the EHR. Certain measures may also provide bonus points, for example, *Query of Prescription Drug Monitoring Program (PDMP)* for Schedule II opioid drugs.

FRAGMENTATION OF ELECTRONIC HEALTH RECORDS AND GETTING THEM TO COMMUNICATE

There are more than 700 federally certified EHR vendors in the United States, with Epic, Cerner, and Meditech combined covering approximately 36% of the market share. In one study of EMR vendors at hospitals, an average of 16 different EHR vendors were used at any one hospital, with nearly 75% of hospitals dealing with 10 or more outpatient vendors. The use of EHRs and getting different EHRs to communicate and exchange data has been an ongoing effort that has been on the federal agenda for decades. In fact, in President George W. Bush's State of the Union Address in 2004, he stated, "By computerizing health records, we can avoid dangerous medical mistakes, reduce costs, and improve care." In 2009, the HITECH Act passed by President Obama led to a $35 billion expenditure to promote and expand the adoption and use of EHRs by eligible hospitals and health care professionals. Five years later in 2014, the Argonaut Project was launched to create a standard protocol for EHR systems to communicate, which ultimately led to the development of the Fast Healthcare Interoperability Resource (FHIR). Today in 2019, nearly 96% of hospitals use some form of EHR, but interoperability is still in its infancy.

For all stakeholders, this significant level of fragmentation has led to a push for creating standardized protocols of communication as well as interface engines that can help transfer data in a bidirectional manner. For physicians, the multitude of EHR systems likely means memorizing multiple different passwords, multiple different ways to access one patient's data, and inefficiencies across multiple workflows. Take one clinical scenario as an example. If a patient with a hand infection presents to the hand surgeon's office, this will mean using the outpatient office EHR, ordering laboratory tests to be done at another location (perhaps by paper order), sending the patient to the phlebotomy office that will likely have a completely separate EHR system, and then waiting for a paper fax with laboratory results to come back to the hand surgeon's office. If the patient then requires surgery, perhaps the patient will need to see his or her medical doctor for medical optimization and clearance. This may introduce another separate EHR system, and the hand surgeon's office will then likely receive the clearance note by PDF or fax. Finally, once the patient has surgery, documentation of this surgery may actually occur in a separate system if the location of the surgery has a different EHR. Thus, in 1 clinical scenario, 4 separate systems may potentially be invoked without any digital overlap across the differing EHRs.

For patients, the isolation of data in any one system can create significant delays in their care. For example, in another common clinical scenario, a patient who presents to an outside urgent care center with a wrist fracture will likely have no direct way of transferring his or her images, reports, or documents to the hand surgeon. Similarly, if a new patient presents to the hand surgeon's office after having received care in a separate hospital system or another physician's office, the patient will likely have to reregister, repeat input of his or her medical history, medications, and other information, along with possible duplication of medical imaging. If advanced imaging (eg, MRI or computed tomography scan) was performed, this would then require an authorization of release from one institution to another and potentially create another delay of care.

Electronic interface engines are designed to help communicate between EHRs using cross-platform standards. One commonly used set of standards is HL7 (Health Level Seven International), which defines and provides a framework for data exchange, decision support, syntax rules for clinical documents, quality reports, prescription medications, and other clinical information. HL7 includes several different standards to cover different functions, including the following:

- HL7 Messaging Version 2 and 3, which is currently the most widely used messaging standard for exchanging clinical information
- C-CDA (consolidated-clinical document architecture), an exchange model for clinical documents (eg, discharge summaries and progress notes), which is also associated with CCD (Continuity of Care Document) that details patient discharge and admission among separate facilities
- FHIR, one of the most recent efforts to leverage API technology to help communicate information between EHRs

FHIR has quickly become the newest focus for interoperability among EHRs. It differs from prior standards because it moves away from the older paradigm of document exchange, and instead focuses on exchange of more discrete information using Web-based technology. For instance, instead of transferring whole documents, such as an entire progress report or discharge summary, FHIR would use unique addresses for discrete information, such as the care plan, medications, or family history. This discrete information could then be pulled into any application using their unique address, similar to a URL for a Web site, and the information could be recompiled into a document. Although FHIR has taken over the EHR industry as a new standard recently, full implementation will likely require much more time.

LEVERAGING ADVANCED FEATURES

The EHR can also enhance the practice of hand surgery in ways that are less commonly discussed. For example, as a database of patients and patient demographics, the EHR can provide insight for significant analysis. Here are just a few examples of leveraging data from the EHR to help advance your practice:

- *Analysis of patient population.* Routine or intermittent analysis of where patients reside can help direct marketing toward certain regions or local neighborhoods with lower rates. This information also can contribute to downstream development decision making, for example, if the practice is considering opening satellite offices, or branching out with urgent care locations.
- *Analysis of payer mix and referral sources.* It also may be helpful to analyze the regions by payer mix as well as by method of patient referrals. Some EHRs may allow entry of discrete data regarding the referring physician; this may come in the form of specific individuals or clinicians (eg, primary care doctors), or type of referral (eg, physical therapist, chiropractor, primary care doctor, neurologist). Leveraging these data may identify opportunities for targeted growth and expansion. Combined with collection and revenue data, it also may be possible to calculate average revenue per patient, which may then be used in a variety of models to help with practice management considerations.
- *Internal analysis of utilization.* In a growing practice, the EHR also can help with improving workflow efficiency. For example, a hand surgeon who is beginning a practice may find it useful to track and analyze numbers of filled and empty appointment slots before considering hiring physicians extenders, such as medical assistants, physician assistants, or a scribe. As the hand surgeon's practice matures, it also may be more efficient to develop templates for the office schedule that outlines when New patients, Postoperative patients, and Follow-up patients are allowed to book their appointments. Spacing these appointments

appropriately can help with efficiency for multiple staff members. For example, new patients who may require radiographs can be booked so they do not overlap with postoperative patients who may also require radiographs. Alternatively, if a medical assistant or physician assistant usually performs a new patient intake, these may be spaced apart from postoperative appointments if they also require the attention of these personnel for removal of sutures or take down of dressings and splints.

DISCLOSURE

The authors have nothing to disclose.

REFERENCES

1. Office-based Physician Electronic Health Record Adoption. Available at: https://dashboard.healthit.gov/quickstats/pages/physician-ehr-adoption-trends.php. Accessed September 29, 2019.
2. Garrett P, Seidman J. EMR vs EHR – What is the Difference?. 2011. Available at: https://www.healthit.gov/buzz-blog/electronic-health-and-medical-records/emr-vs-ehr-difference. Accessed September 29, 2019.
3. Evans RS. Electronic health records: then, now and in the future. Yearb Med Inform 2016;(Suppl1):S48–61.
4. Institute of Medicine. The computer-based patient record: an essential technology for health care. In: Dick RS, Steen EB, Detmer DE, editors. Revised edition. Washington, DC: National Academy Press; 1997.
5. Marquez G. The history of electronic health records (EHRs). 2017. Available at: https://www.elationhealth.com/clinical-ehr-blog/history-ehrs/. Accessed September 29, 2019.
6. Shultz CG, Holmstrom HL. The use of medical scribes in health care settings: a systematic review and future directions. J Am Board Fam Med 2015;28(3):371–81.
7. Montague E, Asan O. Dynamic modeling of patient and physician eye gaze to understand the effects of electronic health records on doctor-patient communication and attention. Int J Med Inform 2014;83:225–34.
8. Asan O, Montague E. Technology-mediated information sharing between patients and clinicians in primary care encounters. Behav Inf Technol 2014;33:259–70.
9. Koshy S, Feustel PJ, Hong M, et al. Scribes in ambulatory urology practice: patient and physician satisfaction. J Urol 2010;184:258–62.
10. Arya R, Salovich DM, Ohman-Strickland P, et al. Impact of scribes on performance indicators in the emergency department. Acad Emerg Med 2010;17:490–4.
11. Bank AJ, Obetz C, Konrardy A, et al. Impact of scribes on patient interaction, productivity, and revenue in a cardiology clinic: a prospective study. Clinicoecon Outcomes Res 2013;5:399–406.
12. Allen B, Banapoor B, Weeks E, et al. An assessment of emergency department throughput and provider satisfaction after the implementation of a scribe program. Adv J Emerg Med 2014;517319.
13. Quality payment program. Available at: https://qpp.cms.gov/mips/overview. Accessed October 5, 2019.
14. Transitions of care. Available at: https://www.healthit.gov/test-method/transitions-care. Accessed October 5, 2019.

Physician Reimbursement
Fee-for-Service, Accountable Care, and the Future of Bundled Payments

Anne J. Miller-Breslow, MD[a],*, Noah M. Raizman, MD, MFA[b]

KEYWORDS

- Bundled payments • MACRA • Physician reimbursement

KEY POINTS

- The fee-for-service model of physician reimbursement based on relative value units has gone unchanged for several decades and is currently under scrutiny.
- The passage of the Patient Protection and Affordable Care Act formalized previously voluntary quality metrics and accountable care requirements.
- Bundled Care Payment Initiatives (BCPI) are gaining traction as a means to lower costs. Under BCPI, payments use a set fee based on an episode of care.
- While attempting to diminish the incentives for volume-based reimbursements, the potential impact on care for patients with higher risks has not yet been determined, nor have the potential cost savings been realized.

INTRODUCTION—A BRIEF HISTORY OF PHYSICIAN REIMBURSEMENT IN THE UNITED STATES

Before 1992, physicians in the United States were paid on a fee-for-service (FFS) basis using the usual and customary rate (UCR), a set of values determined by commercial insurance companies and not disclosed to practitioners. Patients paid the physician directly, and those who had insurance could submit a copy of the bill to the insurer who would then reimburse the policy holder based on the UCR.

FFS also applied to patients over 65 years via the Medicare system. Enacted in 1965 under the Social Security Act during the Presidency of Lyndon Johnson[1] Medicare enrollment began in 1966. The system was administered by the Bureau of Health Insurance, a government entity that, as of 1977, became the Health Care Financing Administration (HCFA). Before 1966 there was no coverage for people over 65 years unless their

workplace had provided insurance as a retirement benefit. Although procedures were documented using a preliminary form of the CPT (Common Procedural Terminology) codes, reimbursement was not yet tied to procedural coding.

Given the opacity of the UCR, there was a perception that its use was not accurate in properly gauging physician work and thus compensation. A group of public health researchers at Harvard Medical School were tasked with determining the relative values of procedures and care rendered by physicians, formulating the concept of the resource-based relative value unit (RVU).[1,2] Their intent was to quantify the relative amount of work performed during a procedure or episode of care, valued by time, intensity, difficulty, resource utilization, and risk.

Their methodology of assigning RVUs to a procedure, based on the results of surveys asking physicians to provide a rank order within a family of procedures, was adopted by HCFA in 1992 and has been the basis for reimbursement since

[a] Englewood Hospital Medical Center, Englewood, NJ, USA; [b] The Centers for Advanced Orthopaedics, 1015 18th Street NS, Suite 300, Washington, DC 20036, USA
* Corresponding author. 151 West 86th Street, New York, NY 10024.
E-mail address: AnneJMiller@icloud.com

Hand Clin 36 (2020) 189–195
https://doi.org/10.1016/j.hcl.2019.12.002
0749-0712/20/© 2019 Elsevier Inc. All rights reserved.

that time. The commercial insurance companies have used the same system of RVUs to determine their rates of reimbursement as this was perceived to be a substantial improvement over the previous UCR system.[2] The use of CPT codes to document the procedures performed has been codified since the 1990s and remains in use by both commercial and government insurers.

THE VALUE OF A RELATIVE VALUE UNIT

The relative value of a CPT code as of 2020 is based on a combination of physician work (approximately 50.9%) and practice expense (44.8%).[3] The physician work takes into account the amount of time, including the procedure as well as preoperative and postoperative care. In addition, the needed technical skill and physical effort as well as the level of stress and potential risk to the patient are included in the value of an RVU. The practice expense component is modified based on a formula that takes the site of service into account. This component is meant to compensate physicians for the administrative costs of patient care. In addition, a professional liability insurance factor accounts for 4.3% of the total value. Each year the Centers for Medicare and Medicaid Services (CMS) determines a monetary conversion factor, which is then used to turn the amount of an RVU within a CPT code into a payment amount.

Although incredibly complex in the details, the bird's eye view of physician reimbursement has been very straightforward over the past 3 decades. A particular procedure or patient encounter (whether in the office, emergency room, or hospital) is associated with a specific CPT code, which is then submitted for reimbursement to the insurer. The values are based on the RVUs for each code with payments then determined by CMS or by the commercial insurer. Commercial insurance companies have used the CMS rates as the basis for their own reimbursements.[4] Therefore, any changes in the Medicare system will also be seen across multiple insurers.

Although hospital payment for an episode of care is billed and reimbursed separately from that of the treating physician, the 2 payees are often closely related. CMS reimbursement to hospital inpatient facilities is based on a diagnosis-related group (DRG), wherein each patient is placed into a category based on diagnosis or surgical procedure and comorbidities, and a lump sum is distributed to the hospital based on the normative data for expected cost of treatment. Commercial payors typically use a similar system. This episode of care-based reimbursement model rewards optimization of length of stay and resource utilization. Concern remains that this model promotes provision of less care and avoidance of sicker patients, given the lack of increased reimbursement for increased services.

RECENT DEVELOPMENTS IN THE HEALTH CARE LANDSCAPE

The costs of medical care have increased over the past several decades, and now account for more than 17% of the GNP,[5] with a significant increase expected over the next decade to more than $6 trillion.[6] This places the United States at the very high end of spending relative to other developed countries, with life expectancy and general health at the lower end.[6] Direct physician reimbursement remains a small portion of the overall health care expenditure, and the number of health care administrators has increased at a rate that dwarfs that of physicians. Yet physician reimbursement remains a target for savings. Initiatives targeted at cost containment and improving the overall value of health care delivered have been the focus of governmental action in recent years.

The methodology of physician reimbursement was changed substantially with the passage of the US Patient Protection and Affordable Care Act (PPACA) in 2010. When studied nationally across medical specialties, the system of FFS has been shown to favor volume over quality, perhaps leading to an overuse of services. To maintain quality and limit costs, an emphasis on cooperation and coordination of care was emphasized.[7] One of the provisions of this new legislation was the creation of the Innovation Center at CMS. This new agency was charged providing Alternative Payment Models (APMs). The most widely known APM initiative has been Bundled Payments for Care Improvement (BPCI).[8]

The earliest federal program focused on quality measures and patient outcomes was the 2007 Physician Quality Reporting Initiative (PQRI). Initially a voluntary program, this early attempt to emphasize quality measures was not adopted by most physicians. The passage of PPACA changed this. PQRI became the Physician Quality Reporting System (PQRS), which subsequently mandated physician participation in the reporting of quality measures and the meaningful use of an electronic health record (EHR) system. The provisions of the PPACA also promoted the formation of affiliated groups and Accountable Care Organizations. A RAND study, sponsored by the American Medical Association in 2015, looked at the effects of the PPACA on physicians.[9] They found that there were shifts in organizational structure with a move toward the formation of large groups as well as hospital affiliations with the idea of cost sharing for the investments in data infrastructure as well as a sense of safety in numbers for negotiations with payors.

This system changed yet again with the passage of the Medicare Access and CHIP Authorization Act (MACRA) in 2015. Before MACRA, the sustainable growth rate (SGR) formula, which had been legislated in 1997 to allow for the federal dollars allotted to Medicare and Medicaid to match the budget, mandated severe and across the board cuts in Medicare payments. Each year it was necessary for Congress to bypass the SGR formula to prevent significant cuts in physician reimbursement. MACRA effectively eliminated the SGR as a threat to physicians.[10]

The Quality Payment Program under MACRA also established the Merit-based Incentive Payment System (MIPS) with an alternative of signing on to an Advanced APM.[11] Their stated goal was to increase the percent of Medicare payments tied to an APM to 30% by 2018 and for those still using FFS the goal was for an 85% tie in to quality or value measures by 2018.[12] MIPS replaced the previously used measures of PQRS, Value Modifiers, and meaningful use of EHR incentives to use electronic prescribing. A new set of monetary rewards and fines were instituted increasing to ±9% over the course of several years. All physicians were mandated to participate unless they had very small volume practice or they were part of an Advanced APM. The practitioners were to be judged on Quality, Resource Use, Clinical Practice Improvement, and Advancing Care Information to come up with a MIPS score, which is then used to determine any potential monetary reward or penalty.

An Advanced APM is an alternative to qualify under MACRA. There are set criteria in regard to becoming a qualified provider under an APM that includes the mandated use of a certified EHR as well as payment by the APM based on quality measures. Specified shared financial risk also needs to be demonstrated. A qualifying provider could be eligible for a 5% lump payment to be paid 2 years after the qualifying year with potential increases in the fee schedule in the future. Although the Advanced APM offers some improvements over previous iterations, little is known currently about its effectiveness in promoting quality care at lower cost. Criticism of MIPS as well as previous iterations of CMS quality measure reporting programs has been the lack of relevance of many quality measures to specialty practice, the burden of data collection, and the lack of consistency of CMS demands over the last decade leading to confusion and increased administrative costs without any demonstrated effect on the quality of delivered care.

As of 2019 there are further proposed changes to the MIPS process entitled MIPS Value Pathways. These pathways attempt to streamline the collection of data, including patient-reported outcome measures and quality measures that are meaningful to physicians' practices and lead eventually to higher value care with a reduced reporting burden.

BUNDLED PAYMENTS: AN ALTERNATIVE MODEL FOR REIMBURSEMENT

Bundled payment is an increasingly popular value-based reimbursement model whereby a single payment is given to a bundle originator ("awardee") to encompass a defined episode of care. Some models focus only on inpatient care, whereas other models include preoperative care, physician reimbursement, inpatient care, postacute care, and subsequent follow-up care, including ancillary therapy, medications, and medical equipment.

In the United States, this concept was first tested for coronary artery bypass grafting at the Texas Heart Institute.[8] Significant cost savings were achieved. Several Centers of Excellence created bundled care pilot programs from 1991 to 1994. In 2009, CMS initiated a preliminary experiment with bundled care in 5 health systems for an acute care episode with a single payment, including physician and hospital reimbursement. In 2013, CMS expanded bundled payments through the BPCI program, which was voluntary. Four separate models were proposed by CMS, with "Phase 1" pilot programs to demonstrate feasibility followed by progression to a "Phase 2" expansion.

Model 1 defined the episode of care to the inpatient stay only, with physician fees continued in the FFS model. Model 2, the most relevant for orthopedic/hand care, includes the inpatient stay, the postacute care, and all additional services up to 90 days from hospital discharge. Model 3 is focused on rehabilitation services, skilled nursing facilities, and long-term care hospitals. In models 2 and 3, reimbursement is still provided using an FFS model (ie, physicians still submit claims), but reimbursements are later reconciled against the bundled payment amount and any overage is then recouped by CMS. Model 4 includes only the inpatient stay, but provides a single payment, which is then distributed by the hospital directly, with providers not submitting separate claims.

A planned mandatory expansion for total joint replacement, termed Comprehensive Care for Joint Replacement was proposed in 2016 but later canceled.[13] At present, participation remains voluntary.

As of July 2018, the voluntary BPCI initiative had 1025 participants in Phase 2, of which 192 were physician group practices, 255 were acute care hospitals, and the rest split between rehabilitation, nursing, and long-term care facilities.[14] A total of 432 of the participants were in model 2, representing all of the physician groups and most of the acute care facilities. Only 48 potential episodes of care were selected by CMS for BPCI. Those potentially relevant to hand and upper extremity surgeons include the DRGs that encompass amputations, procedures involving the humerus, upper extremity joint replacement, arthropathies, sprains/strains/dislocations, tendonitis, and removal of orthopedic devices. However, if BPCI is expanded to include other DRGs, these may become relevant to hand surgeons also.

The most recent evaluation of the BPCI program (October 2018)[15] noted that model 2 accounted for nearly 90% of the episodes, most of which were hip and knee replacements. Medicare payments declined for most clinical episodes in model 2, typically related to decreased use of postacute care (ie, skilled nursing or rehabilitation facilities). Quality of care, measured by emergency room visits, mortality, and readmissions, did not decline significantly. BPCI reconciliation payments for performance to providers offset the cost savings and the overall outcome was a small net loss to Medicare. The CMS report notes that for 2 model 2 episodes—joint replacement and cervical fusion—patients selected for BPCI were less resource intensive than the baseline, indicating that healthier patients were likely to have been cherry-picked for bundles to give the appearance of cost savings.

Successful bundling requires the coordination, alignment, and cooperation of several entities that had previously been reimbursed with an FFS model independently of one another. Appropriate price-setting for the bundle is critical, given the risk for underuse of needed care, leading to poor outcomes if the price is set too low or lack of incentive for efficiency and cost savings if too high. Outlier high-cost cases can lead to significant losses for awardees, and patients with severe complications may be denied care to avoid exposure to costly treatment that exceeds the bundle price.

Given the various legal challenges to the PPACA and the inherently political and shifting nature of leadership in the Department of Health and Human Services, which oversees CMS, the future of the BPCI program remains in flux. Currently, although most care episodes saw some degree of savings, this was offset by performance incentives. With little evidence of overall savings, the appetite for widespread expansion of bundled payments on the part of both government and commercial payors is questionable, although research continues and commercial payors contintue to explore bundled payment.

BUNDLED PAYMENTS: LESSONS FROM TOTAL JOINT ARTHROPLASTY

Several lessons can be gleaned from the early literature on bundled payments for total knee and hip arthroplasty. Concerns for poor outcomes because of disincentivizing therapy utilization and other resources do not seem to be well founded. There was some concern that healthier patients with fewer comorbidities were selected for bundles, given that participation has been voluntary, but there may also be a tendency for better preoperative management of comorbidities to lessen their impact to the bundled episode of care.[16] The early results of BPCI for inpatient total joint replacement are a decreased overall length of stay and a higher discharge to home versus a skilled nursing facility or subacute rehabilitation facility.[17,18] Economic analysis shows that the surgery itself is the largest driver of cost.[19] There is significant concern that bundled payments may compromise access to care for sicker, more comorbid, or vulnerable patients, although there is no evidence of this.[20] Total costs for knee replacement are significantly higher in more complicated patients[21] as well as in older and frailer patients,[22] and these factors predict costs exceeding bundled payment targets.[23] Consequently, risk stratification and adjustment of bundles to account for comorbidities may be necessary to protect vulnerable populations.

Cost savings in the model 2 bundle have been based largely on decreased utilization of postacute care facilities[15,17] At present, BPCI does not allow bundling for outpatient procedures, even outpatient total joint replacement. Beyond the decrease in the use of postacute care facilities, it remains unclear where additional cost savings will occur. One potential for lower expenditures is increasing pressure on implant manufacturers to provide lower cost implants. Although this may only affect the implant companies' margins, it can also have a stifling effect on innovation and lead to smaller sales forces and poorer service.

A potential race to the bottom for facilities to lower their costs will likely only occur if the bundle awardee is not the facility itself. The possibility for physicians and other service providers to be forced to accept decreased reimbursements also exists, particularly in situations where the awardee is the hospital system. In the setting of employed providers, these decreased reimbursements can be offset by overall profitability of the facility. In any case, whoever "owns the bundle" is incentivized to decrease utilization of resources outside their control and increase the proportion of services provided by the awardee and its employees.

Commercial bundles may allow the bundling of outpatient procedures in the future. Given the often less-cohesive nature of outpatient surgery, with multiple independent providers of acute and postacute services, coordination, incentivization, and participation remains uncertain and would likely rely on an independent convener to administer the bundle, potentially providing an entirely new level of administration.

BUNDLING HAND SURGERY: ARE THERE OPPORTUNITIES?

At present, the BPCI has only proposed bundles for a small number of DRGs potentially related to hand surgery. There are currently no data from CMS that can be specifically related to the bundling of hand surgical procedures, and the often outpatient nature of hand surgery means that bundles may have to be reconceptualized to begin either with preoperative diagnosis or outpatient surgery to capture the appropriate episode of care. Unlike total joint replacement, there are often multiple injuries being treated or multiple procedures performed in 1 episode, confounding efforts to establish a bundled value for an episode of care based on the outpatient equivalent of a single DRG. There are currently no bundled payment programs proposed by CMS that address these issues.

There are several potential targets for bundled payments in hand surgery, with distal radius fractures (DRFs) being studied in most detail. Huetteman and colleagues[24] found that the average cost for care of a DRF undergoing open reduction and internal fixation (ORIF) was $7286, with 86% of the cost of treatment attributed to the surgical cost itself. They noted that the variation in postoperative costs was small but that the cost of surgery varied substantially. Kazmer and colleagues[25] examined direct costs associated with DRF ORIF and found that implant manufacturer, number of plates and screws, and hospital versus ambulatory setting were the factors most highly associated with increased costs. In addition, they found that open fractures were more expensive, but that

fracture severity did not independently lead to higher direct costs.

The implication of these studies is that the surgery itself has highly variable costs that may be subject to optimization and efficiency were a DRF bundle to be proposed. Implant costs are substantial and, although pressure may reduce markups, there likely exists a floor beyond which savings are minimal. Several studies have suggested that the use of postoperative occupational therapy does not significantly change outcome[26,27] but, given the low proportion of overall cost attributable to postoperative management, it seems unlikely that use of postoperative therapy is a driver of cost that would lead to increased savings. Godfrey and colleagues[28] evaluated the costs of treating pediatric DRFs and found that, in a large academic center, cost variation was minimal. They hypothesized that their low cost variability made DRF well suited for bundling.

Successful bundling in hand surgery will likely rely on creating reproducible evidence-based guidelines or care maps to reduce variability in resource utilization and costs. With the increase in wide awake local anesthesia as an alternative to regional or general anesthesia for many hand cases, additional potential savings in overall costs may be possible. As literature emerges on the safety of office-based procedures with field sterility, procedural costs associated with draping, equipment, staffing, and disposables may also decline.

A major concern for bundled care is that, in the current system, the bundle begins with either hospitalization or surgery. Substantial cost savings are possible if evidence-based guidelines are used to control unnecessary imaging, diagnostic tests, and therapeutic modalities before specialist consultation and establishment of a definitive treatment plan. The logistics of incorporating primary care and emergency care into a bundled episode of care become increasingly complicated—merely defining the diagnosis that triggers the bundle is problematic, and if primary care practitioners originate a bundle based on presumptive diagnosis and control subsequent access to specialist care, it may be increasingly difficult for a patient to receive appropriate evaluation by a hand surgeon.

THE FUTURE: STAKEHOLDER ALIGNMENT

Current bundled payment initiatives proposed by CMS have been focused on overall cost savings, and early results suggest that quality of care can be maintained, but there is likely a floor beyond which savings are possible. With multiple potential bundle awardees, ranging from hospitals to physician groups to health systems that own hospitals and employ physicians as well as manage ancillary staff, many scenarios involve stakeholders competing for a limited number of dollars. For bundled payment systems and other forms of alternative payment to thrive without having a negative effect of physician reimbursement, stakeholders need to be aligned to find efficiencies and optimize care. This will likely hinge on the use of evidence-based practice guidelines, care maps, and other care optimization tools, especially those that recognize cost-effectiveness as a parameter. High-level informatics will be necessary to demonstrate value and quality of care, and the widespread adoption of EHR systems will facilitate this.

DISCLOSURE

The authors have nothing to disclose.

REFERENCES

1. Hsiao WC, Braun P, Dunn D, et al. Resource-based relative values. An overview. JAMA 1988;260(16): 2347–53.
2. Hsiao WC, Braun P, Dunn DL, et al. An overview of the development and refinement of the resource-based relative value scale the foundation for reform of U.S. physician payment. Med Care 1992; 30(Supplement 1):NS1-12.
3. American Medical Association. RVS update process 2019. Chicago: American Medical Association; 2020.
4. Clemens J, Gottlieb JD. In the shadow of a giant: Medicare's influence on private physician payments. J Polit Econ 2017;125(1):1–39.
5. Papanicolas I, Woskie LR, Jha AK. Health care spending in the United States and other high-income countries. JAMA 2018;319(10):1024.
6. Keehan SP. National health expenditure projections. Health Aff 2012;2019:2019–21.
7. Thorpe KE, Ogden LL. Analysis and commentary. The foundation that health reform lays for improved payment, care coordination, and prevention. Health Aff (Millwood) 2010;29(6):1183–7.
8. Delisle DR. Republished: big things come in bundled packages: implications of bundled payment systems in health care reimbursement reform. Am J Med Qual 2019;34(5):482–7.
9. Friedberg MW, Chen PG, White C, et al. Effects of health care payment models on physician practice in the United States. Rand Health Q 2015;5(1):8.
10. Manchikanti L, Helm Ii S, Calodney AK, et al. Merit-based incentive payment system: meaningful changes in the final rule brings cautious optimism. Pain Physician 2017;20(1):E1–12.
11. MIPS Alternative Payment Models (APMs)—QPP. Available at: https://qpp.cms.gov/apms/mips-apms. Accessed September 19, 2019.
12. Centers for Medicare & Medicaid Services (CMS), HHS. Medicare Program; Merit-Based Incentive Payment System (MIPS) and Alternative Payment Model (APM) Incentive under the physician fee schedule, and criteria for physician-focused payment models. Final rule with comment period. Fed Regist 2016;81(214):77008–831.
13. CMS finalizes changes to the comprehensive care for joint replacement model, cancels episode payment models and cardiac rehabilitation incentive payment model | CMS. Available at: https://www.cms.gov/newsroom/press-releases/cms-finalizes-changes-comprehensive-care-joint-replacement-model-cancels-episode-payment-models-and. Accessed September 29, 2019.
14. Bundled Payments for Care Improvement (BPCI) Initiative: General Information | Center for Medicare & Medicaid Innovation. Available at: https://innovation.cms.gov/initiatives/Bundled-Payments. Accessed September 19, 2019.
15. The Lewin Group. CMS Bundled Payments for Care Improvement (BPCI) initiative models 2-4: year 4 evaluation & monitoring. Annual Report October, 2018. p. 174.
16. Plate JF, Ryan SP, Black CS, et al. No changes in patient selection and value-based metrics for total hip arthroplasty after comprehensive care for joint replacement bundle implementation at a single center. J Arthroplasty 2019;34(8):1581–4.
17. Haas DA, Zhang X, Kaplan RS, et al. Evaluation of economic and clinical outcomes under centers for medicare and medicaid services mandatory bundled payments for joint replacements. JAMA Intern Med 2019;179(7):924.
18. El-Othmani MM, Sayeed Z, Ramsey JA, et al. The joint utilization management program—implementation of a bundle payment model and comparison between year 1 and 2 results. J Arthroplasty 2019. https://doi.org/10.1016/j.arth.2019.06.041.
19. Navathe AS, Troxel AB, Liao JM, et al. Cost of joint replacement using bundled payment models. JAMA Intern Med 2017;177(2):214.
20. Maughan BC, Marrufo G, Kahvecioglu DC. Bundled payments for hospitals: the authors reply. Health Aff 2019;38(7):1230.
21. Anis HK, Sodhi N, Vakharia RM, et al. Cost analysis of medicare patients with varying complexities who underwent total knee arthroplasty. J Knee Surg 2019. https://doi.org/10.1055/s-0039-1695716.
22. Pepper AM, Novikov D, Cizmic Z, et al. Age and frailty influence hip and knee arthroplasty reimbursement in a bundled payment care improvement initiative. J Arthroplasty 2019;34(7):S80–3.

23. Ryan SP, Goltz DE, Howell CB, et al. Predicting costs exceeding bundled payment targets for total joint arthroplasty. J Arthroplasty 2019;34(3):412–7.

24. Huetteman HE, Zhong L, Chung KC. Cost of surgical treatment for distal radius fractures and the implications of episode-based bundled payments. J Hand Surg Am 2018;43(8):720–30.

25. Kazmers NH, Judson CH, Presson AP, et al. Evaluation of factors driving cost variation for distal radius fracture open reduction internal fixation. J Hand Surg Am 2018;43(7):606–14.e1.

26. Souer JS, Buijze G, Ring D. A prospective randomized controlled trial comparing occupational therapy with independent exercises after volar plate fixation of a fracture of the distal part of the radius. J Bone Joint Surg Am 2011;93(19):1761–6.

27. Chung KC, Malay S, Shauver MJ, et al. The relationship between hand therapy and long-term outcomes after distal radius fracture in older adults. Plast Reconstr Surg 2019;144(2):230e–7e.

28. Godfrey JM, Little KJ, Cornwall R, et al. A bundled payment model for pediatric distal radius fractures. J Pediatr Orthop 2019;39(3):e216–21.

Evidence-Based Hand Therapy and Its Impact on Health Care Policy

Lesley Khan-Farooqi, OTD, OTR, CHT[a],*, Ekta Pathare, FACHE, MBA, OTR, CHT[b]

KEYWORDS

- Evidence-based medicine • Advocacy • Health policy • Systematic reviews • Collaboration
- Partnerships • Hand therapy • Reimbursement

KEY POINTS

- The unique and collaborative relationship between hand therapists and surgeons is invaluable in meeting the unique functional needs of clients with upper extremity conditions and injuries.
- Current legislative issues and research items that directly affect hand therapy and hand surgery practice include the opioid epidemic, the importance of optimizing function, value-based care, and the expansion of evidence-based medicine to support clinical decisions.
- This calls for the need for hand therapists to develop and use evidence that can drive policy change and optimize outcomes for clients with upper extremity conditions and injuries.

INTRODUCTION

In today's rapidly changing health care environment, collaborative care and partnerships can optimize client care to advance common goals in practice, research, and legislation.[1] The collaborative relationship between hand therapists and hand surgeons is invaluable in meeting the unique needs of clients with upper extremity conditions. The art and science involved in both hand therapy and surgery requires specialized skills to prevent upper limb dysfunction, restore function, and potentially reverse pathologic conditions to allow clients to participate in everyday activities.[2]

BATTLING THE OPIOID EPIDEMIC

One of the biggest political accomplishments this past year was the advancement in legislation to battle the opioid epidemic. Clients with acute and chronic pain can face significant challenges physically, emotionally, and financially. The Pain Management Best Practices Inter-Agency Task Force (Task Force) was developed to identify best practices for managing acute and chronic pain. The strategies identified included the importance of patient-centered care in diagnosis and treatment and having measurable outcomes that show improvements in quality of life and function.[3]

The Task Force recognizes the value of a comprehensive pain management team, often requiring the integration of various health professionals who work together on a multidisciplinary team to achieve excellence in patient-centered care. The alliance between health professionals including hand surgeons and hand therapists, who consist of both occupational therapists and physical therapists, can address the complex aspects of pain, including the bio-psychosocial effects of the unique needs of upper extremity clients. Evidence supports that a coordinated and multidisciplinary approach can reduce pain and improve overall quality of life and function.[4]

Often pain is the primary reason that clients with upper limb musculoskeletal disorders (MSDs) are referred to a hand therapist.[5] Current evidence

[a] Occupational Therapy Program, University of St Augustine, 5401 La Crosse Avenue, Austin, TX 78613, USA;
[b] CGAIT Global LLC, ASHT, Education Committee, ACHE of North Texas, 841 Crestview Drive, Coppell, TX 75019, USA
* Corresponding author.
E-mail address: lkhan-farooqi@usa.edu

Hand Clin 36 (2020) 197–203
https://doi.org/10.1016/j.hcl.2020.01.005

supports the importance of addressing not only the underlying physical components of the injured or degenerated tissue but also the client's unique psychosocial factors. Pain is a subjective experience that is unique to each individual client because of the interactions of biological, psychological, and social factors.[5] Psychological factors that can affect pain and disability association with an MSD include cognitive, affective, and behavioral factors.[6,7]

Cognitive factors associated with pain affect how an individual perceives potential or actual nociceptive stimuli. Pain self-efficacy, which is a sense that one will be able to manage the pain he or she may experience, has been associated with someone experiencing less pain and having better function.[5] Pain catastrophizing is an exaggerated negative response to actual or anticipated pain and is associated with feelings of helplessness, increased pain, and disability.[5] Therefore, reducing pain catastrophizing and increasing pain self-efficacy is an approach therapists and physicians apply to reduce experienced pain and increase function.

The Task Force recognizes the importance of restorative therapies including occupational therapy and physical therapy. It also recognizes that allied health professions often face challenges with reimbursement policies. To overcome these challenges, the Task Force suggests research to support restorative therapies as part of a multidisciplinary approach. These restorative approaches include the use of therapeutic exercise, manual therapy, and therapeutic modalities such as transcutaneous electrical nerve stimulation, superficial and deep heat modalities, and cryotherapy.

FOCUSING ON FUNCTIONAL PARTICIPATION

As part of the educational standards, both occupational and physical therapy students are required to demonstrate proficiency in the delivery of therapeutic exercise and therapeutic modalities.[8,9] These therapeutic approaches have been regularly used in hand therapy practice, but in recent years there has been a bigger emphasis on the importance of practicing occupation-based therapy.[10] Occupation-based activities have been at the core of occupational therapy practice since its conception in 1917.[11] The recent shift in occupation-based interventions in literature has been driven by the World Health Organization (WHO) and the International Classification of Functioning, Disability and Health (ICF), which includes terms such as activity and participation. These terms are defined as a "task or action by an individual" and "involvement in a life situation,"

respectively. As the ICF provides a standard language and framework for all health professionals, this calls for a focus on function in both the occupational and physical therapy professions.[10]

The definition of occupation-based interventions does vary within the literature, but there is a general agreement that a therapeutic functional activity could be a simulated or actual life task of the client. The use of occupation-based interventions has the ability to be more engaging and automatic for clients to complete, thus facilitating their participation and distracting them from the pain or anxiety they may be experiencing during their recovery process.[10] In a systematic review, Weinstock-Zoltnick and Mehta[10] found that overall, clients who engaged in occupation-based therapy had better outcomes in patient-related, performance, and physical measures of the upper extremity. Thus, the unique art and science of hand therapy and surgery call for an occupation-based approach to ensure functional use of the upper quadrant.

EXPANSION OF EVIDENCE-BASED MEDICINE

Recent legislation promoted by the US Department of Health and Human Services and National Institutes of Health (NIH) emphasize the importance of rehabilitation research to promote participation and function.[12] The National Center for Medical Rehabilitation Research led the development of the NIH Plan for Rehabilitation Research, which outlines a plan to conduct and coordinate medical rehabilitation research through the NIH. The research agenda supports research on the following topics:

- Understanding the pathophysiology and management of nervous and musculoskeletal conditions
- Understanding the appropriate timeline for rehabilitative interventions
- Understanding and refining evidence-based rehabilitation strategies
- Developing best practices for pediatric rehabilitation
- Understanding secondary conditions that may be associated with chronic disabilities
- Developing of orthotics, prosthetics, and other technologies or devices that support function

The current research plan is due to be updated in 2021 as required by the 21st Century Cures Act.[13]

The National Institute of Arthritis and Musculoskeletal and Skin Diseases (NIAMS) under the NIH supports research specifically for causes, treatment, and prevention of conditions of the bones, joints, muscles, and skin.[14] In 2019, the appropriations amount for NIAMS was US$605,065,000 with an adjusted President's budget of $520,829,000 in 2020. Recent research initiatives by NIAMS have focused on basic science research for new therapeutic interventions, biomedical science including the identification of biomarkers, and the development of transformative tools and technologies.[14] These funding opportunities have the potential to directly facilitate the outcomes of clients.

VALUE-BASED CARE

A recent shift in health care is the push for value-based care from volume-based care. With the 2019 Physician Fee Schedule (PFS) final rule, there is a shift to focusing on improving client care coordination, health outcomes, and streamlining processes. Physicians and other health care professionals have struggled with the time constraints of completing excessive regulatory requirements and paperwork, which can interfere with direct patient care time. This initiative has been referred to as "Patients over Paperwork" to allow physicians to spend time on patient care rather than the completion of excessive documentation.[15] Clear and concise documentation is important for physicians to focus on providing quality care and receive timely reimbursement for services.

A major change in documentation includes the ability to focus on functional status changes, rather than re-recording information that has already been documented in the client's medical record. Previous client information should be reviewed by the practitioner and updated as appropriate.[15] Coding and reimbursement will now be based on the client's history, examination, and medical decision making (MDM). This will allow physicians to spend time counseling, educating, and coordinating the necessary care for their clients by billing for their time and MDM.[15] This change can have a significant impact in the area of upper extremity surgery where time is necessary to appropriately counsel clients and coordinate care with other health professions, including occupational and/or physical therapy.

Another change from the PFS that could have an impact on upper extremity surgery and rehabilitation is the use of virtual care. The 2020 and 2019 PFS both recognized the importance of technology in health care. These advances include reimbursement for the use of virtual checkins and remote evaluation of patient-submitted photos or videos.[15] In addition, virtual care can also play a role in prolonged preventative care services and services for opioid use or substance use disorders.

IMPACT ON THERAPY SERVICES

A major change to therapy reimbursement will occur because of the Bipartisan Budget Act of 2018. As a result of the Bipartisan Budget Act of 2018, a reduction in reimbursement for occupational therapy assistants (OTAs) and physical therapy assistants (PTAs) will take effect in 2022.[16] OTAs and PTAs will be reimbursed at a rate of 85% of the PFS rate for occupational and physical therapy services. As of January 1, 2020 occupational therapists working in outpatient settings will need to use the modifier CO, whereas physical therapists working with outpatients will use modifier CQ to document when therapy services are furnished all or in part by a therapy assistant.[16] The CY20 Proposed Rule has the same requirement, but also will require additional documentation to justify whether the modifier was applied or not applied. The concern for hand therapists is that these additional documentation requirements may become burdensome and take away the priority of patient care. In addition, the CY20 Proposed Rule would apply a 10% de minimis standard to determine when the reduction in reimbursement will be applied. The Centers for Medicare and Medicaid Services (CMS) proposes that therapy services furnished by greater than 10% of the total service by an OTA or PTA will require the application of the modifier.[16]

QUALITY PAYMENT PROGRAM

The Quality Payment Program (QPP) was introduced in 2017 to promote the quality of patient care and improved patient outcomes. There are 2 options to participate, the Merit-Based Incentive Payment System (MIPS) and Advanced Alternative Payment Models. The main objective of QPP is to improve the quality of patients' care and their outcomes by rewarding participating clinicians.[17] When the MIPS program initially started there was flexibility in the participation criteria, with a performance threshold that increased overtime. This flexibility provided to clinicians did result in an overall high rate of participation, with 98% of eligible clinicians participating in 2018. However, improvements are still needed within the MIPS program.[17]

Areas of potential improvement for MIPS in the future include decreasing the complexity and improving the clarity of performance requirements. This feedback led to the Patients over Paperwork initiative to streamline the requirements and reduce clinician burden.[15,17] The number of MIPS quality measures were also reduced to ensure that the included measures were high-quality and meaningful to improving patient care. The CMS is proposing MIPS Value Pathways (MVPs), which would apply to proposals that begin in the 2021 performance year.[17]

The MVPs initiative focuses on aligning measurement options that are relative to the clinician's scope of practice while also being applicable to providing quality patient care. This program would look to align measures and activities within the MIPS performance categories: Quality, Cost, Promoting Interoperability, and Improvement Activities. Through this program a clinician or group would be in one MVP that is associated with their specialty or with a condition they commonly treat, thus reporting the same measures and activities as other clinicians or groups within that MVP.[17] This program would also look to reduce the reporting burden by limiting the number of specialty or condition-specific measures, to allow clinicians to report on the same measurement set(s).

LEGISLATIVE IMPACT AND MOVING FORWARD

The process of evidence-based hand therapy influencing health care policy offers tremendous opportunity. Synthesizing evidence to inform policy makers becomes the professional responsibility of all hand therapists. Rising health care costs create challenges for resource allocation and legislative decisions. Legislative impact is a collaborative approach between hand therapy professionals, surgeons, professional societies, advocacy groups, professional regulating organizations, state organizations, researchers, evidence-based networks, and policy makers.[18]

BARRIERS IN DECISION MAKING

Literature review indicates that not many policy makers perform systematic reviews or meta-analysis when shaping health care policy. Decisions are influenced by legal issues, public opinion, stakeholder interests, financial implications, and existing IT systems. Policy makers may not find it possible to read or access appropriate journal articles or possess skills to appraise and interpret clinical research or be able to search through overwhelming volumes of available research.[18] Any one discipline or its members lack complete knowledge of the change process, thus policy making is a transdisciplinary approach. Election cycles, policy making, and research often occur at different times, causing a time mismatch barrier. Evidence also changes with time and as new information becomes available. Researchers lack time and personal contact with policy makers.[19]

BEST PRACTICES IN IMPLEMENTATION

Data-driven decision making is becoming increasingly possible with digitization. The WHO uses Evidence Briefs for policy, based on local research and systematic reviews and policy dialogs between policy makers and researchers. They also use rapid-response services to provide resources at short notice to policy makers. A bigger goal is also to increase awareness and knowledge about the link between evidence and policy, thus leading the policy-making culture to be evidence based. Dialog, exchange of ideas, and sharing of information, ideas, and opinions help to promote knowledge transfer.[20]

IMPLEMENTATION

Hand therapists could use a systematic approach. The first step is to identify a problem, following which the hand therapist should seek evidence and take steps to define the problem. The WHO provides a systematic overview of the change process. Defining the problem is followed by defining the solution. Using a data-driven and analytical approach provides support toward implementing a successful policy change. Quality screening is an essential step toward identifying options and policy implementation considerations. Conducting ongoing dialog and nurturing relationships ensures a sustainable policy change and implementation[20] (**Fig. 1**). Advocacy efforts and Legislative Action Centers of professional organizations offer ways to voice concerns, share opinions, and learn other therapists' perspectives.

EVIDENCE TYPE

Policy-making evidence should include quantitative data and qualitative accounts. Quantitative evidence typically includes scientific information and data from peer-reviewed journals, systematic reviews, analytical data from administered programs, surveys, single studies and evaluations, collective opinions and professional perspectives, and statistical information. Qualitative evidence can be in the form of compelling stories and narrative accounts, non-numerical observations, persuasive stories, and occurrences as examples.[21]

EVIDENCE-BASED POLICY SYSTEMS

Evidence-based policy making occurs in incremental progression and is inherently a complex process. It is worthwhile for hand therapists to understand methods that can increase the probability of policy change. Studies have found that advocacy efforts by leaders and professional experts in collaboration with research

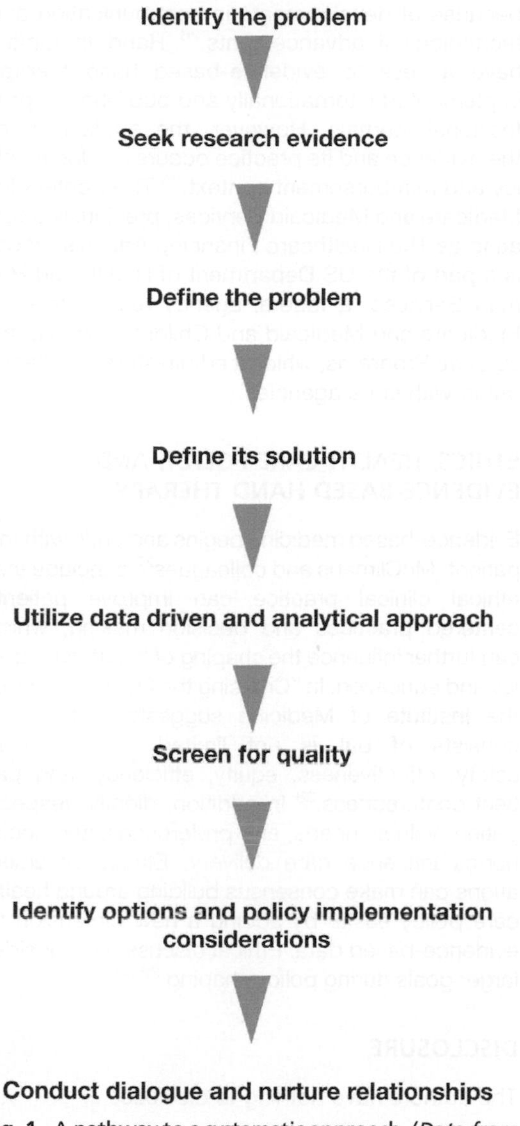

Identify the problem

Seek research evidence

Define the problem

Define its solution

Utilize data driven and analytical approach

Screen for quality

Identify options and policy implementation considerations

Conduct dialogue and nurture relationships

Fig. 1. A pathway to a systematic approach. (*Data from* World Health Organization. EVIPNet in action - Executive Summary. World Health Organization 2016.)

and well-grounded scientific findings influence policy. In addition, social marketing, persuasive issue articulation, political factors, and cost-benefit comparisons represent tools that can aid with policy formulation.[21]

A review of literature from political science revealed that numerous factors including political, social, financial, and administrative factors, among others, affect a government's decision to implement policy. Actions that are considered and weighed during policy formulation can include:

- Evaluating available solutions
- Conducting a cost-benefit analysis to possible actions

- Assessing the possible effects the actions will have on the health group
- Conducting comparisons between equitable and recommended policy types being considered
- Considering political costs and system change costs associated with various options
- Identifying various advocacy groups involved and being affected by the policy changes, their value systems, their influences, their strategy, and their frames of reference[22]

Hand therapists should take these factors into consideration before making their case. Policy, once implemented, can be continuously monitored and evaluated to assess expected versus actual outcomes. Assessment can include relevance to current research, health care research, and possibilities for further improvement, or even complete removal of the policy.

A comprehensive understanding of the US government health care policy formulation system is essential for a hand therapist. Although professional associations and ethics groups are largely involved in policy making, the next few lines elaborate on the government component of policy formulation. In his essay, Gostin[23] provides insight on the legally binding and law-enforced official policy making, which comprises:

- Executive
- Legislature
- State and Federal Judiciary levels

Various task forces, advisory entities, trade associations, professional organizations, public interest, consumer- and community-based groups, and presidential and congressional commissions influence and provide information toward the making of policy. Impartial decision making, complying with a fair process, displaying accountability, and considering and accumulating complete objective information are key components of a good decision-making process. Of the 3 branches, the legislature and executive are the most suited for policy decision making and have the ability to gather data and information from a wide variety of sources. Barriers to sound decision making at the legislature level can be a result of politically influenced leaders serving as decision makers, individual ideologies, competing interests between organizations and groups, and the collective influence that members of large associations and organizations can have on election results. These can inherently cause biases in sound policy formulation. The executive branch being best situated can access data and evidence in the form of clinical, policy research, public health, prevention, and financial impact information from the NIH, Agency for Health Care Policy and Research, Centers for Disease Control and Prevention, and The Centers for Medicare and Medicaid Services.[23]

ROLE OF ADVOCACY

Advocacy and advocacy groups can play the role of bridging the gap between researchers and policy makers. Policy makers are rarely medical professionals and may have a slim understanding of patient treatments and needs. Policy formulations occur at organizational, state, regional, and federal levels. Leadership and informed advocacy skills will aid a hand therapist to communicate effectively with stakeholders at all levels of governance.

Professional organizations and societies provide a platform for professionals with similar interests and goals to come together toward a common purpose. Organizations become stronger with the numerical representation of their membership, and advocacy efforts can lead to collective success especially when represented in large numbers.[24] Organizations offer tools for advocacy and enormous research literature to enable policy change and education of stakeholders and policy makers. Professional associations influence policy making through collective effort and expertise of its individual members and formulations of practice guidelines. It affords transparency to perspectives, experiences, professional judgments, and data assessment. Policy making is hugely affected by individual experiences, expertise, and judgments of policymakers.[25]

FINANCIAL IMPACT

Evidence-based policy may imply that decision makers use data, information, research and evidence and conduct a systematic analysis of available research before making reimbursement policy decisions and developments. Before the new policy decisions are made, economic and research evidence are considered in addition to the cost-effectiveness and therapeutic value added in terms of quality of life and functional gains. Decision making considers value added in comparison with cost to society. Negotiations between stakeholders, despite the presence of scientific data, contribute significantly on how health care is delivered. Considering diminishing resources and budgetary constraints, financial considerations are a major factor in evidence-based policy development and formulation.[25] Increased health care spending does not always correlate with better health. Worldwide data and scientific knowledge have become easily available

because of developments in communication and technological advancements.[26] Hand therapists have access to evidence-based hand therapy implemented internationally and published in professional journals. However, the application of the evidence and its practice occurs in a local policy and reimbursement context.[26] The Centers for Medicare and Medicaid Services, previously operating as The Healthcare Financing Administration, is a part of the US Department of Health and Human Services, a federal agency responsible for Medicare and Medicaid and Children's Health Insurance Programs, which it administers in collaboration with state agencies.

ETHICS, HEALTH CARE POLICY, AND EVIDENCE-BASED HAND THERAPY

Evidence-based medicine begins and ends with the patient. McClimans and colleagues[27] conclude that ethical clinical practice can improve patient-centered practices and decision making, which can further influence the shaping of health care policy and education. In "Crossing the Quality Chasm," the Institute of Medicine suggests that quality consists of but is not limited to timeliness, safety, effectiveness, equity, efficiency, and patient-centeredness.[28] In addition, dignity, respect, patient values, needs, and preferences, and social norms influence care delivery. Ethical considerations can make consensus building around health care policy easier by adding a new dimension to evidence-based data. Ethical discussions consider larger goals during policy shaping.[29,30]

DISCLOSURE

The authors have nothing to disclose.

REFERENCES

1. Moyers PA, Metzler CA. Health policy perspectives—interprofessional collaborative practice in care coordination. Am J Occup Ther 2014;68:500–5.
2. Hand Therapy Certification Commission. Definition of hand therapy. 2019. Available at: https://www.htcc.org/consumer-information/the-cht-credential/definition-of-hand-therapy.
3. Health and Human Services. Pain management best practices inter-agency task force report: updates, gaps, inconsistencies, and recommendations. 2019. Available at: https://www.hhs.gov/sites/default/files/pain-mgmt-best-practices-draft-final-report-05062019.pdf.
4. Stanos S. Focused review of interdisciplinary pain rehabilitation programs for chronic pain management. Curr Pain Headache Rep 2012;16(2):147–52.

5. Hamasaki T, Pelletier R, Bourbonnais D, Harris P, Choiniere M. Pain-related psychosocial issues in hand therapy. J Hand Ther 2018;31:215–26.

6. Vranceaunu AM, Barsky A, Ring D. Psychosocial aspects of disabling musculoskeletal pain. J Bone Joint Surg Am 2009;91(8):2014–8.

7. Schindeler P, Stegink-Jansen CW. Introduction: psychosocial issues at hand. J Hand Ther 2011;24(2):80–1.

8. American Occupational Therapy Association. 2018 Accreditation council for occupational therapy education (ACOTE®) standards and interpretive guide. 2018. Available at: https://www.aota.org/~/media/Corporate/Files/EducationCareers/Accredit/Standards Review/2018-ACOTE-Standards-Interpretive-Guide.pdf.

9. American Occupational Therapy Association. Physical agent modalities. Am J Occup Ther 2012;62:691–3.

10. Weinstock-Zoltnick G, Mehta S. A systematic review of the benefits of occupation-based interventions for patients with upper-extremity musculoskeletal disorders. J Hand Ther 2018;32(2):141–52.

11. American Occupational Therapy Association. AOTA's centennial vision and executive summary. Am J Occup Ther 2007;62:613–4.

12. U.S. Department of Health and Human Services. The National Center for Medical Rehabilitation Research (NCMRR). 2019. Available at: https://www.nichd.nih.gov/about/org/ncmrr. Accessed July 27, 2019.

13. American Occupational Therapy Association. AOTA advocates for rehabilitation research as NIH develops 5-year research plan. Available at: https://www.aota.org/Advocacy-Policy/Congressional-Affairs/Legislative-Issues-Update/2019/AOTA-Advocates-for-Rehab-Research.aspx. Accessed July 27, 2019.

14. National Institute of Arthritis and Musculoskeletal and Skin Diseases. FY 2019 funding plan 2019. Available at: https://www.niams.nih.gov/about/budget/fy2019. Accessed August 6, 2019.

15. Centers for Medicare and Medicaid Services. Calendar Year (CY) 2019 Medicare physician fee schedule (PFS) final rule. Available at: https://www.cms.gov/About-CMS/Story-Page/CY-19-PFS-Final-Rule-PPT.pdf. Accessed September 12, 2019.

16. Centers for Medicare and Medicaid Services. Physician fee schedule. Available at: https://www.cms.gov/Medicare/Medicare-Fee-for-Service-Payment/Physician FeeSched/. Accessed September 30, 2019.

17. Centers for Medicare and Medicaid Services. Quality payment program proposed rule overview factsheet with request for information for 2021 2020. Available at: https://qpp-cm-prod-content.s3.amazonaws.com/uploads/594/2020%QPP%20Proposed%20Rule%20Fact%20Sheet.pdf. Accessed September 12, 2019.

18. Bunn F, Sworn K. Strategies to promote the impact of systematic reviews on healthcare policy: a systematic review of the literature. Evidence Policy 2011;7:403–28.

19. Brownson RC, Chriqui JF, Stamatakis KA. Table 1. Am J Public Health 2009;99(9):1577. Available at: https://www.ncbi.nlm.nih.gov/pmc/articles/PMC2724448/#!po=8.33333.

20. World Health Organization. EVIPNet in action—executive summary. Geneva: WHO; 2016.

21. Brownson RC, Chriqui JF, Stamatakis KA. Understanding evidence-based public health policy. Am J Public Health 2009;99(9):1576–83.

22. Benoit F. Public policy models and their usefulness in public health: the stages model. Montreal (Quebec): National Collaborating Centre for Healthy Public Policy; 2013.

23. Gostin L. The formulation of health policy by the three branches of government. In: Bulger RE, Meyer Bobby E, Fineberg HV, editors. Society's choices: social and ethical decision making in biomedicine. Washington, DC: National Academies Press (US); 1995. p. 335–57. Available at: https://www.ncbi.nlm.nih.gov/books/NBK231979/.

24. Kristine A, Huynh BS, Chung KC. Concepts of organizational excellence in medical associations. Plast Reconstr Surg Glob Open 2019;7:e2300.

25. Van Herck P, Annemans L, Sermeus W, et al. Evidence-based health care policy in reimbursement decisions: lessons from a series of six equivocal case-studies. PLoS One 2013;8(10):e78662.

26. Clancy CM, Cronin K. Evidence-based decision making: global evidence, local decisions. Health Aff (Millwood) 2005;24(1):151–62.

27. McClimans LM, Dunn M, Slowther A. Health policy, patient-centred care and clinical ethics. J Eval Clin Pract 2011;17(5):913–9.

28. Committee on Quality of Health Care in America, Institute of Medicine. Crossing the quality chasm: a new health system for the 21st century. Washington, DC: National Academy Press; 2001.

29. Danis M Clancy CM Larry R.Ethical dimensions of health policy.Oxford University Press.New York

30. Ruger JP. Ethics in American Health 1: ethical approaches to health policy. Am J Public Health 2008;98(10):1751–6.

Access to Hand Therapy Following Surgery in the United States
Barriers and Facilitators

Jasmine Krishnan, OTRL, CHT, MHSA, BSc(H)OT[a],*, Kevin C. Chung, MD, MS[b]

KEYWORDS

- Postoperative therapy • Hand therapy • Rehabilitation • Therapy access

KEY POINTS

- Outcomes after hand surgery can be dependent on delivery of postoperative hand therapy services.
- Access to hand surgery does not guarantee access to hand therapy.
- Several factors influence a patient's ability to receive hand therapy.
- Ongoing efforts are needed to preserve and improve access to hand therapy following hand surgery.

BACKGROUND

Hand therapy is an essential component of postoperative care for many hand conditions.[1–3] The Triple Aim consists of improving patient experience, improving health, and reducing per capita health care costs.[4] Meeting this aim requires cohesive teamwork among the hand surgeon, hand therapist, and patient.[5] In alignment with this model, hand therapy serves to maximize functional outcomes through timely progression of postoperative rehabilitative protocols.[5] This includes management of edema, early detection of complications, and timely identification of need for interventions such as psychological counseling. Effective hand therapy reduces cumulative costs by limiting the duration of rehabilitation, the patient's time off work, and the possible need for future surgical interventions. Cost-effectiveness and cost-utility analyses have become prevalent tools in calculation of value of health care expenditure.[6] As a result, hand therapy can be important in informing health policy pertaining to hand surgery, including reimbursement policies.

Hand therapy in the United States is provided by a state licensed occupational therapist (OT) or physical therapist (PT).[7] A certified hand therapist (CHT) is an OT or a PT who has earned certification from the Hand Therapy Certification Commission (HTCC) after passing a test on advanced clinical skills and theory in upper quarter rehabilitation.[8] In this article, we collectively refer to OTs and PTs treating patients who have undergone hand surgery as "hand therapists," and OT and PT services as "hand therapy" or "therapy" unless intentionally differentiated.

Initiation of hand therapy, following a formal referral from a hand surgeon, commences an episode of care that is specific to the International Classification of Diseases, Tenth Revision, Clinical Modification (ICD-10-CM) code that is descriptive

[a] Michigan Medicine, Rehabilitation Services, Domino's Farms, Lobby A, Plastic Surgery Suite, Room 1108, 24 Frank Lloyd Wright Drive, SPC 5735, Ann Arbor, MI 48106, USA; [b] Michigan Medicine, Section of Plastic Surgery, University of Michigan Medical School, 1500 East Medical Center Drive, 2130 Taubman Center, SPC 5340, Ann Arbor, MI 48109-5340, USA
* Corresponding author.
E-mail address: jasminek@med.umich.edu

Hand Clin 36 (2020) 205–213
https://doi.org/10.1016/j.hcl.2020.01.006
0749-0712/20/© 2020 Elsevier Inc. All rights reserved.

of the patient's injury or related diagnosis.[9] The recommended number of visits in each episode of care and its duration are unique to each patient and informed by the following:

- Complexity of injury and/or repair
- Postoperative rehabilitative protocols
- Recovery and/or postoperative complications
- Individual patient characteristics, such as functional expectations
- Ability to follow instructions for a home exercise program

Occupational therapy and physical therapy are 2 exclusive allied health professions that are reimbursed for delivery of care independently of one another and of physicians. Reimbursement is also separate from hospitals if care is delivered in an outpatient setting. Therapy services are billed following a standard format under the Healthcare Common Procedure Coding System (HCPCS). This assigns a unique procedural code for each service provided to the patient, irrespective of reimbursement structure.[10] Therapy is billed as a time-based service using HCPCS Level I Current Procedural Terminology (CPT) in increments of 15 minutes.[10,11] Single unit charges are submitted for non–time-based services, such as application of a heat pack or use of paraffin. Supplies and materials, including orthoses, are billed using HCPCS Level II codes.[10] Outpatient OT and PT services are reimbursed under fee-for-service or percentage of charges payment methods.[12]

Most CHTs practice in outpatient settings that are the focus of discussion in this article.[13] However, in the presence of complex hand trauma or comorbidities that delay discharge of patients to independent community living, initial hand therapy may be provided in acute care hospitals, acute inpatient rehabilitation hospitals, subacute rehabilitation facilities, or home health care settings. Owing to the need for staff who can treat a multitude of medical conditions, access to specialized hand therapists may be limited in these scenarios. These instances of care are largely reimbursed under a per episode, per diem payment or discounted rate methodology by Medicare and other payers.[12] On the other hand, outpatient therapy coverage for medically insured individuals is a vast and variable conglomerate of insurance plans, each one of them unique in its specifications of coverage and limitations.[14] In this article, we discuss the factors that facilitate and hinder access to outpatient hand therapy (**Figs. 1** and **2**). In addition, several promising initiatives are explored.

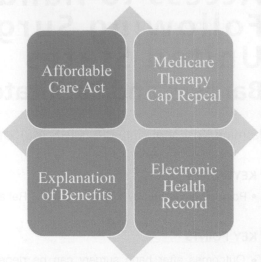

Fig. 1. Facilitators for access to hand therapy.

FACTORS FACILITATING ACCESS TO HAND THERAPY AFTER HAND SURGERY
Patient Protection and the Affordable Care Act: Ten Essential Health Benefits

After passage of the Patient Protection and Affordable Care Act (ACA), the number of uninsured nonelderly adults decreased from 44 million in 2013 to 27 million in 2016.[15] Signed into law in 2010, and effective in 2014, the ACA mandates health insurance entities to provide coverage of 10 essential health benefits, including rehabilitative and habilitative services, such as hand therapy.[16] Toker and colleagues[17] present evidence of better adherence to hand therapy and superior outcomes following flexor tendon repair in patients with insurance coverage for postoperative rehabilitation. Therefore,

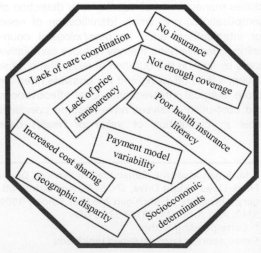

Fig. 2. Barriers against access to hand therapy.

expansion of insurance coverage may increase access and improve effectiveness of hand surgery.

The ACA also eliminates increased premiums or refusal to provide coverage based on preexisting conditions.[16] This facilitates access to hand therapy for those who undergo secondary surgeries after hand trauma and corrective or reparative surgeries for progressive conditions, such as rheumatoid arthritis. However, effective 2019, the federal government announced discontinuation of federal penalty for voluntary refusal to obtain health insurance without an exemption.[18] This policy change may influence the number of uninsured patients in need of hand therapy.

Regulatory Actions

Federal and state health care regulations are in constant flux and affect patients' access to hand therapy. Two examples are listed as follows:

- In 1997, the Centers for Medicare and Medicaid Services (CMS) introduced an annual expenditure cap on outpatient therapy services for Medicare beneficiaries.[19] Patients who underwent complex hand surgery were put at a disadvantage, especially those who underwent multiple hand surgeries or sustained unrelated medical problems requiring therapy within a single calendar year. Occasionally, in the absence of exceptions processes, rationing of visits for much-needed and time-sensitive hand therapy was the only choice.[19] On February 9, 2018, the Bipartisan Budget Act of 2018 that repealed application of the Medicare outpatient therapy expenditure cap was signed into law. This is a monumental step in favor of access to hand therapy for patients who require extended rehabilitation after surgery.[20]
- On January 12, 2017, CMS withdrew a proposed rule that would require a provider to have specified qualifications and accreditation to bill for prostheses and custom fabricated orthoses.[21] If passed, it would have limited hand therapists' ability to fabricate custom orthoses for Medicare beneficiaries.[21] Custom orthoses, uniquely designed to protect surgically repaired structures, are often one of the first interventions that hand therapists provide to enable progression of postoperative mobilization protocols. Withdrawal of this proposal has preserved hand therapists' ability to provide this service.

Patient Access to Explanation of Benefits

Insurance companies provide an explanation of benefits (EOB) to inform beneficiaries of plan discounts, charges reimbursed to medical providers, and patients' financial responsibilities per encounter.[22] Some insurance companies provide electronic access to EOBs to improve timely access to this information.[23,24] Financial information from past visits might not reflect the exact costs of future visits. It can, however, provide some estimate. This is important for patients receiving hand therapy because their cost is a sum of uncovered portions of charges for each visit, and not one lump sum share of a bundled rate (**Table 1**).

Electronic Health Record

According to the Office of the National Coordinator for Health Information Technology (ONC), as of 2017, 96% of all hospitals have adopted Certified Electronic Health Record Technology, and 86% of office-based physicians have adopted the basic electronic health record (EHR).[25,26] Evidence on whether electronic medical records assist in care coordination is still inconclusive, and gaps remain in its development to promote interorganizational communication.[27] However, the EHR has improved communication within organizations.[27] The EHR can improve operational efficiency and ensure timely access to hand therapy. It also provides multi-user application with simultaneous access for health care providers and ancillary team members. This assists in prompt identification of referrals from hand surgeons and timely initiation of administrative processes, such as obtaining insurance verification prior to scheduling appointments. In addition, access to detailed medical records can provide valuable information to the therapist regarding surgery and comorbidities. This informs sound clinical reasoning and professional judgment. The EHR also enhances communication between surgeons and therapists, which is essential for patient safety.

Table 1 Cost sharing for outpatient hand therapy can be a recurring expense	
Hand Therapy Visits	**Patient Cost per Visit**
#1	$ a
#2	$ b
#3	$ c
#4	$ d
#5	$ e
Total patient cost = $(a + b + c + d + e)	

BARRIERS TO HAND THERAPY ACCESS AFTER HAND SURGERY

No Health Insurance

The number of uninsured nonelderly adults decreased from 2013 to 2016; however, the uninsured population increased by 700,000 in 2017, to 27.4 million. This was the first increase since the implementation of ACA.[15] According to Henry Kaiser Family Foundation, 45% of uninsured nonelderly adults cited high cost, whereas 22% cited loss of job as the primary reason for remaining uninsured in 2017.[15] Changes in health policy influence access to health care coverage, which in turn determines whether or not a patient will receive assistance in paying for hand therapy. Impact analyses of the repeal of individual mandate penalty under the ACA that went into effect in 2019 indicate that insurance premiums would have been lower without this repeal.[28] Increasing premiums might result in an increase in the number of uninsured adults. Patients who are uninsured are expected to assume uncertain financial responsibility because of inadequate price transparency in outpatient services.[29] This deters patients from committing to therapy. It also should be noted that uninsured individuals are often charged more than what third-party payers pay.[15]

Inadequate Insurance Coverage for Hand Therapy

Hand therapy visits are recurring and may take place anywhere from 1 to 5 times a week in the initial postoperative period. Allied health supervisor and CHT at Michigan Medicine, Ms Carole Dodge, stated that many health insurance plans impose a limit on the number of occupational therapy or physical therapy visits allowed per diagnosis per year and may also limit the duration of an episode of care. Most third-party payers have processes in place to request extension of hand therapy visits beyond allowed limits, but contractual agreements are seldom overridden. Restricted coverage of therapy sessions can affect patients' ability to adhere to essential protocols in the initial stages of rehabilitation.[17] They run the risk of exhausting allowed visits before progressing to later stages of therapy. Patients in this situation are prone to rationing their therapy visits, which leads to poorer health outcomes.

Poor Health Insurance Literacy

Besides high premiums, lack of health insurance literacy has been identified as a barrier to appropriate insurance coverage selection.[30] Older adults with inadequate health insurance literacy

may not be able to identify important attributes of available Medicare Advantage plans, which can result in reduced access to health care and higher costs.[31] Commercial plans offer cost-sharing options, such as copay, coinsurance, and deductible. However, such terms are not well understood and can be a significant source of confusion for patients.[32,33] Some health insurance companies have made efforts to educate their members on common terms, but it is unclear how many beneficiaries have a clear understanding before selecting plans.[34,35] As of 2016, research indicated that adequate information regarding rehabilitative coverage is lacking in the Summary of Benefits and Coverage.[36] Consumers use this resource to make informed decisions on selection of coverage plans under the ACA.[36]

Consumers must be well informed before choosing insurance. An example of recent changes in support of need for increased health insurance literacy is presented by the issuance of the Short Term Final Rule by the Department of Health and Human Services.[37] Effective October 2, 2018, this policy allows coverage under short-term plans for up to 364 days that may be extended for up to 36 months.[37] Concern from this ruling arises from the exemption of short-term plans from having to adhere to the ACA requirements, specifically the coverage of all essential benefits, including rehabilitative services and coverage of preexisting conditions.[38] Individual states are responding variably to this ruling, and there is concern that patients might not be able to afford and will therefore decline much-needed therapy services.[38]

Increasing Cost Sharing by Consumer

Enrollment in High Deductible Health Plans (HDHPs) in the United States increased from 2007 to 2017, among adults aged 18 to 64, with employment-based coverage.[39] HDHPs offer lower premiums than traditional plans but carry a higher out-of-pocket deductible and may be combined with a Health Savings Account.[40] No specific studies appear to have evaluated the impact of HDHPs on utilization of hand therapy. However, there are studies indicating that those enrolled in HDHPs with chronic conditions bear increasing financial burdens and are likely to delay or decide against obtaining essential medical services.[41,42] Systematic reviews have indicated that HDHPs reduce utilization of health care.[43] There is concern that HDHPs will result in greater barriers to hand therapy access for low-income families. This opinion is based on studies reporting the higher financial burden of HDHPs that may lead individuals to delay or forgo care.[44,45]

Geographic Disparity in Provider Access

Contact information of CHTs is available on the HTCC Web site and is searchable by ZIP code, city and state, company, last name, and even country for those who wish to attend hand therapy closer to their residence.[46] However, CHTs are unevenly distributed, and practice only in 9% of the US ZIP Code Tabulation Areas.[47] Most CHTs are located in urban areas with high population density and large health centers, or in smaller centers with strong academic hand surgery presence.[47] This presents a significant obstacle when patients undergo hand surgery far from home but need to attend multiple postoperative hand therapy appointments over extended periods.

Socioeconomic Determinants of Health

Low-income individuals enrolled in Medicaid are not guaranteed access to hand therapy due to variation and sometimes exclusion of occupational therapy coverage in different states and plans.[48] Social, economic, and environmental disadvantages reduce access to health care.[49] Even when insurance pays for therapy, patients may cite inability to take time off from work, childcare, or copays as obstacles to attending therapy. Lack of financial resources also present a challenge to patients who must pay for travel to a distant hand therapist.[50]

Care Coordination in a Siloed Health Care Delivery System

Effective interpersonal and interdisciplinary communication is required to ensure appropriate delivery of health care.[51] Most hand therapy practitioners likely agree that there are opportunities to improve care coordination to facilitate timely access to hand therapy, especially transition of care between facilities. For example, patients are often referred to hand therapists closer to their home, only to return to the original facility weeks later. These patients report an inability to attend therapy elsewhere because of exclusion of their insurance plans or a communication gap between case managers and facilities. It is common for patients to admit to not realizing how important it is to attend hand therapy. Patients in such cases lose precious time in their recovery. This adversely affects outcomes after hand surgery.

Lack of Price Transparency

Are we able to provide a reasonable cost estimate to our patients before they agree to receive hand therapy services? Are we able to provide a breakdown of charged amount, insurance discounts, and remaining patient balance, before providing services? In addition, are we able to provide any definitive information on self-pay discounts? Inability to answer these questions is a barrier against access to hand therapy. Transparency in outpatient pricing is lacking and poses a challenge for patients who share high costs with third-party payers or are uninsured.[29] Patients are unable to obtain estimated cost of services because multiple payer systems have vastly varied benefits.[52] The actual services and time required for hand therapy is also uncertain before initiating an episode of care. A lack of access to this information deprives patients of the resources needed to avoid unexpected financial liability. In addition, it presents a significant deficit in providing transparency as defined by the US Government Accountability Office.[52]

Payment Models Limiting Access to Providers

The American Occupational Therapy Association (AOTA) describes inconsistencies in coverage of occupational therapy across various payers, whether private or public. Providers are strongly encouraged to review contractual restrictions so that they can provide ethical hand therapy services while promoting health insurance literacy in relation to hand therapy.[53] Practices must consider various factors before accepting patients who require postoperative hand therapy.[53] Payers may request that individual therapists join a network of providers.[53] Patients may or may not have an option to opt out of in-network providers and might bear an increased financial burden if they receive services from an out-of-network provider.[53] Providers may be dissuaded from accepting plans that offer lower reimbursement rates. For example, Medicare Advantage plans often reimburse less for therapy services than the traditional Medicare plans.[54] These individual payer nuances directly affect a patient's ability to receive hand therapy from the provider or practice of their choice.

EFFORTS TO IMPROVE ACCESS TO HAND THERAPY AND INFORM HEALTH POLICY
Innovative Delivery Methods

The AOTA defines telerehabilitation as application of evaluation, prevention, diagnostic, and therapeutic services via 2-way or multipoint interactive telecommunication technology.[55] Several studies have suggested efficacy of telerehabilitation for musculoskeletal problems with good health outcomes.[56–59] It offers at least a partial solution to overcoming geographic barriers in the field of hand therapy. The hand is an intricate, delicate structure and parallel recovery of all components is necessary to ensure that patients regain their hand function after surgery. This warrants that patients be treated in-person for a thorough evaluation, orthoses fabrication, soft tissue mobilization, edema control, progression of therapy, and effective carryover to a home program. However, telerehabilitation can be valuable as an adjunct mode of delivery for follow-up visits to monitor progress, review home programs, or make minor changes in treatment.

The AOTA recognizes the need for additional research to determine whether telerehabilitation is an effective and ethical delivery method, in line with practice guidelines and standards set by state licensing bodies.[55] In addition, security concerns and adherence to patient health information protection rules remain a point of opposition as we move forward with telerehabilitation.[55] Ongoing efforts to address these concerns, as well as issues such as portability of licensure and reimbursement guidelines, are likely to inform health policy relevant to hand therapy and telerehabilitation.[60]

Integrated Practice Units

Integrated Practice Units (IPUs) are smaller units within health care organizations that are structured around patients' unique medical conditions.[61–64] They are organized to provide patients with continuous care, including health education, inpatient, outpatient, and rehabilitative care.[61–64] Integration of multidisciplinary team members and assumption of joint responsibility ensures that patients receive quality care in IPUs.[61–64] For patients receiving hand surgery specifically, IPUs can improve access to hand therapy. However, it is important to keep in mind that hand therapy is a continuing service and therefore geographic inaccessibility can be a significant hindrance to IPU effectiveness. Approval processes and organization of IPUs for patients receiving hand surgery requires formal liaison with hand therapists outside the local unit (**Fig. 3**). To sustain a successful

partnership, processes must be in place to monitor patient utilization, outcomes, and experience, so that all associated practitioners provide services in accordance with the goals of the IPU.

Interoperability to Promote Interorganizational Communication

The ONC describes interoperability as the capability of 2 or more systems to exchange health information in a useable format.[65] Interoperability among large health systems and small independent private therapy practices with utilization of the EHR will streamline communication and increase access to hand therapy. However, interoperability at this scale is a long-term goal and lack of standardization presents a challenge.[66] Consistent efforts to optimize online documentation processes will not only improve interoperability, but will also assist in retrieval of data. Trends in adoption of EHRs are encouraging.[26] Cumulative data from the EHR is not only useful for tracking patient progress but also can be a resource when negotiating with payers. In addition, standardized data can inform future research efforts and raise the standards of hand therapy practice. Hand therapy–specific customization is necessary to facilitate improvements in efficiency and effectiveness of communication and documentation.

Research Efforts to Expand Evidence Base

Evidence-based practice is a significant factor in enhancing delivery of hand therapy. It not only promotes adherence to best practices, but also provides important data to justify coverage of hand therapy by third-party payers. For example, patients sometimes experience a lag in receiving authorization for hand therapy after common surgical procedures. If evidence of the usefulness of hand therapy in these situations is conveyed to third-party payers, predetermined adjunct hand therapy authorizations can be established. There has been an increase in occupational therapy

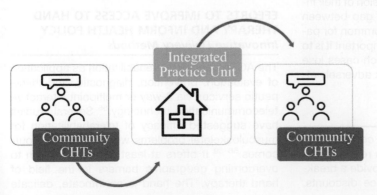

Fig. 3. Liaison of IPUs with CHTs will increase access to hand therapy and add to value for patients.

Integrated Practice Unit

Community CHTs

Community CHTs

doctorate programs, and entry-level physical therapy education has completely transitioned to doctorate programs with an emphasis on evidence-based practice.[67,68] These trends in education will empower practitioners to enhance their evidence-based research efforts.

Improved Organizational Processes

At an organizational level, patients can benefit from processes dedicated to improving care coordination, concentrated on various aspects of hand therapy. For example, policies can mandate that therapy-specific insurance verifications and authorizations be triggered when an elective surgery is scheduled or soon after an unplanned hand surgery. This will result in timely scheduling and provide an opportunity for patients to address limitations in coverage, including cost sharing. Transition to outside facilities also can be addressed ahead of time, which will reduce gaps in care. For efforts to be successful, it is important to develop workflows, dedicated resources, and accountability measures.

SUMMARY

Patients who undergo hand surgery navigate through a fragmented system of multiple providers in various disciplines. Value-based care and reimbursements with emphasis on reporting of outcomes are at the forefront of health care policy changes. Outcome measures that are reflective of collective responsibility and integrated performance of all disciplines in the continuum of care have yet to include hand therapy. Bundled payment models with pay-for-performance methodology might catalyze such change in the future. When that time comes, access to hand therapy will no longer be isolated from hand surgery. Instead, it will be integrated into a seamless continuum of care.

ACKNOWLEDGMENTS

The authors appreciate Carole Dodge, OTRL, CHT, Allied Health Supervisor at Michigan Medicine, Ann Arbor, MI, for providing insight into common limitations in insurance coverage for hand therapy; Jeanne Riggs, OTRL, CHT, Clinical Specialist at Michigan Medicine, Ann Arbor, MI for providing feedback; and Natalie Baxter, Clinical Research Assistant, Section of Plastic Surgery, Department of Surgery, University of Michigan Medical School, Ann Arbor, MI for assistance with editing and illustrations.

DISCLOSURE

The authors have nothing to disclose.

REFERENCES

1. Ray WZ, Mackinnon SE. Clinical outcomes following median to radial nerve transfers. J Hand Surg Am 2011;36(2):201–8.
2. Shores JT, Imbriglia JE, Lee WA. The current state of hand transplantation. J Hand Surg Am 2011;36(11):1862–7.
3. Waljee JF, Chung KC. Objective functional outcomes and patient satisfaction after silicone metacarpophalangeal arthroplasty for rheumatoid arthritis. J Hand Surg Am 2012;37(1):47–54.
4. Berwick DM, Nolan TW, Whittington J. The triple aim: care, health, and cost. Health Aff 2008;27(3):759–69.
5. Mackin EJ. Prevention of complications in hand therapy. Hand Clin 1986;2(2):429–47.
6. Alderman AK, Chung KC. Measuring outcomes in hand surgery. Clin Plast Surg 2008;35(2):239–50.
7. Why see a hand therapist? American Society of Hand Therapists Web site. Available at: https://www.asht.org/patients/why-see-hand-therapist. Accessed June 2, 2019.
8. Who is a certified hand therapist (CHT)? Hand Therapy Certification Commission Web site. Available at: https://www.htcc.org/consumer-information/the-cht-credential/who-is-a-cht. Accessed April 24, 2019.
9. ICD-10 coding. American Society of Hand Therapists Web site. Available at: https://www.asht.org/practice/federalstate-regulations/icd-10-coding. Accessed June 16, 2019.
10. HCPCS codes. American Society of Hand Therapists Web site. Available at: https://www.asht.org/practice/federalstate-regulations/hcpcs-codes. Accessed May 29, 2019.
11. Procedure coding. American Society of Hand Therapists Web site. Available at: https://www.asht.org/practice/federalstate-regulations/medicare/procedure-coding. Accessed May 29, 2019.
12. Quinn K. The 8 basic payment methods in health care. Ann Intern Med 2015;163(4):300–6.
13. Juckett LA, Griffin C. The domains of hand therapy: an inpatient rehab perspective. ASHT Times 2017;24(1):1.
14. Coverage by payer. The American Occupational Therapy Association Web site. Available at: https://www.aota.org/Advocacy-Policy/Federal-Reg-Affairs/Pay.aspx. Accessed July 11, 2019.
15. Key facts about the uninsured population. Henry J Kaiser Family Foundation Web site. 2018. https://www.kff.org/uninsured/fact-sheet/key-facts-about-the-uninsured-population/. Accessed May 7, 2019.
16. Read the Affordable Care Act. Centers for Medicare & Medicaid Services. Available at: https://www.healthcare.gov/where-can-i-read-the-affordable-care-act/. Accessed May 31, 2019.

17. Toker S, Oak N, Williams A, et al. Adherence to therapy after flexor tendon surgery at a level 1 trauma center. Hand 2014;9(2):175–8.

18. No health insurance? See if you owe a fee. Centers for Medicare & Medicaid Services. Available at: https://www.healthcare.gov/fees/fee-for-not-being-covered/. Accessed May 31, 2019.

19. Medicare therapy cap FAQs. American Society of Hand Therapists. Available at: https://www.asht.org/practice/federalstate-regulations/billing. Accessed May 13,2019.

20. Therapy services. Centers for Medicare & Medicaid Services. Available at: https://www.cms.gov/Medicare/Billing/TherapyServices/index.html. Accessed May 13, 2019.

21. Medicare program; establishment of special payment provisions and requirements for qualified practitioners and qualified suppliers of prosthetics and custom-fabricated orthotics; withdrawal. Fed Regist 2017;82 FR 46181:46181–2. Available at: https://www.federalregister.gov/documents/2017/10/04/2017-21425/medicare-program-establishment-of-special-payment-provisions-and-requirements-for-qualified. Accessed June 1, 2019.

22. Understanding your explanation of benefits (EOB). Cigna. 2018. Available at: https://www.cigna.com/individuals-families/understanding-insurance/explanation-of-benefits. Accessed May 31, 2019.

23. How do I read my Blue Cross Blue Shield of Michigan explanation of benefits? Blue Care Network. Available at: https://www.bcbsm.com/index/health-insurance-help/faqs/topics/understanding-benefits/explanation-of-benefits.html. Accessed May 31, 2019.

24. Engage in your health care anytime, anywhere. Aetna. Available at: https://www.aetna.com/individuals-families/health-insurance-through-work/health-insurance-information/tools-and-tech.html. Accessed May 31, 2019.

25. Henry J, Pylypchuk Y, Searcy T, et al. Adoption of electronic health record systems among US non-federal acute care hospitals: 2008-2015. ONC Data Brief 2016;35:1–9.

26. Health IT dashboard. The Office of the National Coordinator for Health Information Technology. 2019. Available at: https://dashboard.healthit.gov/quickstats/quickstats.php. Accessed July 14, 2019.

27. O'Malley AS, Grossman JM, Cohen GR, et al. Are electronic medical records helpful for care coordination? Experiences of physician practices. J Gen Intern Med 2010;25(3):177–85.

28. How repeal of the individual mandate and expansion of loosely regulated plans are affecting 2019 premiums. Henry J Kaiser Family Foundation. 2018. Available at: https://www.kff.org/health-costs/issue-brief/how-repeal-of-the-individual-mandate-and-expansion-of-loosely-regulated-plans-are-affecting-2019-premiums/. Accessed May 31, 2019.

29. Kullgren JT, Duey KA, Werner RM. A census of state health care price transparency Web sites. JAMA 2013;309(23):2437–8.

30. Adepoju O, Mask A, McLeod A. Health insurance literacy as a determinant of population health. Popul Health Manag 2018;21(2):85–7.

31. Braun RT, Barnes AJ, Hanoch Y, et al. Health literacy and plan choice: implications for Medicare managed care. Health Lit Res Pract 2018;2(1):e40–54.

32. Bartholomae S, Russell MB, Braun B, et al. Building health insurance literacy: evidence from the Smart Choice Health Insurance™ program. J Fam Econ Issues 2016;37:140–55.

33. Loewenstein G, Friedman JY, McGill B, et al. Consumers' misunderstanding of health insurance. Am J Health Econ 2013;32:850–62.

34. Explaining premiums, deductibles, coinsurance and copays. Aetna. Available at: https://www.aetna.com/health-guide/explaining-premiums-deductibles-coinsurance-and-copays.html. Accessed May 31, 2019.

35. How do deductibles, coinsurance and copays work? Blue Care Network. Available at: https://www.bcbsm.com/index/health-insurance-help/faqs/topics/how-health-insurance-works/deductibles-coinsurance-copays.html. Accessed May 31, 2019.

36. Analysis of rehabilitation and habilitation benefits in qualified health plans. Stateside Associates. 2016. Available at: https://www.aota.org/Advocacy-Policy/Health-Care-Reform/News/2016/Stateside-Webinar-Analysis-Rehabilitative-Habilitative-Benefits-ACA-Marketplaces-Plans.aspx. Accessed May 28, 2019.

37. Short term, limited duration insurance. The Daily Journal of the United States government. Fed Regist 2018;83 FR 38212:38212–43. Available at: https://www.federalregister.gov/documents/2018/08/03/2018-16568/short-term-limited-duration-insurance#h-3. Accessed May 29, 2019.

38. The short-term plan final rule: what you need to know. The American Occupational Therapy Association. Available at: https://www.aota.org/Advocacy-Policy/Health-Care-Reform/News/2018/Short-Term-Plan-Final-Rule.aspx. Accessed May 29, 2019.

39. Cohen RA, Zammitti EP. High-deductible health plan enrollment among adults aged 18-64 with employment-based insurance coverage. NCHS Data Brief 2018;(317):1–8.

40. High deductible health plan (HDHP). Centers for Medicare and Medicaid Services. Available at: https://www.healthcare.gov/glossary/high-deductible-health-plan/. Accessed June 2, 2019.

41. Galbraith AA, Ross-Degnan D, Soumerai SB, et al. Nearly half of families in high-deductible health plans whose members have chronic conditions face substantial financial burden. Health Aff 2011;30(2):322–31.

42. Galbraith AA, Soumerai SB, Ross-Degnan D, et al. Delayed and forgone care for families with chronic conditions in high-deductible health plans. J Gen Intern Med 2012;27(9):1105–11.

43. Agarwal R, Mazurenko O, Menachemi N. High-deductible health plans reduce health care cost and utilization, including use of needed preventive services. Health Aff 2017;36(10):1762–8.

44. Low-income Americans with employer-sponsored insurance face financial burdens from high-deductible plans. Agency for Healthcare Research and Quality. 2016. Available at: http://www.ahrq.gov/news/newsletters/e-newsletter/545.html. Accessed July 14, 2019.

45. Kullgren JT, Galbraith AA, Hinrichsen VL, et al. Health care use and decision making among lower-income families in high-deductible health plans. Arch Gen Intern Med 2010;170(21):1918–25.

46. Find a CHT. Hand Therapy Certification Commission Web site. Available at: https://www.htcc.org/find-a-cht. Accessed August 11, 2019.

47. Stegink-Jansen CW, Collins PM, Lindsey RW, et al. A geographical workforce analysis of hand therapy services in relation to US population characteristics. J Hand Ther 2017;30(4):383–96.

48. Medicaid. The American Occupational Therapy Association Web site. Available at: https://www.aota.org/Advocacy-Policy/Federal-Reg-Affairs/Pay/medicaid.aspx. Accessed June 2, 2019.

49. Meyer PA, Yoon PW, Kaufmann RB. Introduction: CDC health disparities and inequalities report-United States, 2013. MMWR Suppl 2013;62:3–5.

50. McCarthy ML, Ewashko T, MacKenzie EJ. Determinants of use of outpatient rehabilitation services following upper extremity injury. J Hand Ther 1998; 11(1):32–8.

51. McDonald KM, Sundaram V, Bravata DM, et al. Closing the quality gap: a critical analysis of quality improvement strategies. In: Shojania KG, McDonald KM, Wachter RM, et al, editors. Care Coordination, vol. 7. Rockville (MD): Agency For healthcare research and quality (US); 2007. p. V.

52. Health care price transparency: meaningful price information is difficult for consumers to obtain prior to receiving care. U.S. Government Accountability Office. 2011. Available at: https://www.gao.gov/products/GAO-11-791. Accessed June 3, 2019.

53. Private Pay. The American Occupational Therapy Association. Available at: https://www.aota.org/Advocacy-Policy/Federal-Reg-Affairs/Pay/Private.aspx. Accessed July 14, 2019.

54. Medicare Advantage. American Society of Hand Therapists. Available at: https://www.asht.org/practice/federalstate-regulations/medicare-advantage. Accessed June 17, 2019.

55. Wakeford L, Wittman PP, White MW, et al. Telerehabilitation position paper. Am J Occup Ther 2005; 59(6):656–60.

56. Cottrell MA, Galea OA, O'Leary SP, et al. Real-time telerehabilitation for the treatment of musculoskeletal conditions is effective and comparable to standard practice: a systematic review and meta-analysis. Clin Rehabil 2017;31(5):625–38.

57. Tousignant M, Giguère AM, Morin M, et al. In-home telerehabilitation for proximal humerus fractures: a pilot study. Int J Telerehabil 2014;6(2):31.

58. Moffet H, Tousignant M, Nadeau S, et al. In-home telerehabilitation compared with face-to-face rehabilitation after total knee arthroplasty: a noninferiority randomized controlled trial. J Bone Joint Surg Am 2015;97(14):1129–41.

59. Levanon Y. The advantages and disadvantages of using high technology in hand rehabilitation. J Hand Ther 2013;26(2):179–83.

60. Brown JE. Professional associations, state licensure, and the reimbursement of telerehabilitation. In: Kumar S, Cohn ER, editors. Telerehabilitation. London: Springer; 2013. p. 285–96.

61. Porter ME, Teisberg EO. Redefining health care: creating value-based competition on results. Boston (MA): Harvard Business Press; 2006.

62. van Harten WH. Turning teams and pathways into integrated practice units: appearance characteristics and added value. Int J Care Coord 2018;21(4): 113–6.

63. Lee TH. Discovering strategy: a key challenge for academic health centers. Trans Am Clin Climatol Assoc 2016;127:300.

64. Porter ME. A strategy for health care reform—toward a value-based system. N Engl J Med 2009;361(2): 109–12.

65. Fact Sheets. The Office of the National Coordinator for Health Information Technology. Available at: https://www.healthit.gov/topic/fact-sheets. Accessed June 12, 2019.

66. Shared Nationwide Interoperability Roadmap: The Journey to Better Health and Care. The Office of the National Coordinator for Health Information Technology. Available at: https://www.healthit.gov/infographic/shared-nationwide-interoperability-roadmap-journey-better-health-and-care. Accessed June 12, 2019.

67. Case-Smith J, Page SJ, Darragh A, et al. The professional occupational therapy doctoral degree: why do it? Am J Occup Ther 2014;68(2):e55–60.

68. Physical therapist (PT) education overview. American Physical Therapy Association. Available at: https://www.apta.org/For_Prospective_Students/PT_Education/Physical_Therapist_(PT)_Education_Overview.aspx. Accessed July 07, 2019.

The Intersection of Hand Surgery Practice and Industry

Arnold-Peter C. Weiss, MD[a,b,]*

KEYWORDS

- Industry • Commercialization • Intellectual property • Products • Implants

KEY POINTS

- Interactions between doctors and industry representatives should not exchange anything of value related to use.
- Physicians should strive to use the best equipment, implants, and devices available for each patient's needs regardless of any industry contacts.
- Developing products or services with industry requires disclosure to all, including patients.
- Several key steps are required in the process of sale of intellectual property, licensing of a product or codevelopment to protect all parties.
- Physicians with an inherent conflict of interest in a product or service related to medicine should be careful in public presentations or publication of data related to the former.

INTRODUCTION

The relationship between hand surgeons (or any other physicians) and industry (of any type, including pharmaceuticals, medical device manufacturers, and service providers) generally involves 2 distinct interactions:

- The working relationship between physicians and industry in a daily clinical sense
- The interaction between physicians who wish to be directly involved in product development and their chosen industry partners

Managing conflict of interests, financial relationships, protection of intellectual property, timing of a relationship, consulting versus royalty versus direct sale versus other equity arrangements, and eventual product marketing and sales requires ethics, safeguards, and careful documentation.

CLINICAL PRACTICE CONFLICTS OF INTEREST IN INDUSTRY INTERACTIONS

The American Academy of Orthopaedic Surgeons (AAOS) has an extensive statement of Orthopaedist-Industry Conflicts of Interest in which the following appears: "Orthopaedic surgeons must be mindful of potential conflicts of interest with patient care in pursuing academic and commercial ventures. A conflict of interest exists when professional judgment concerning the well being of the patient has a reasonable chance of being influenced by other interests of the physician. The self-interest of the physician may be financial in nature. The competing interests may involve fame and notoriety for the physician or time for the physician or the physician's family."[1]

In general, hand surgeons may accept minor gifts, medical textbooks, or patient education

a Hand & Upper Extremity Surgery, Department of Orthopaedics, Alpert Medical School of Brown University, Providence, RI, USA; b University Orthopedics, 1 Kettle Point Avenue, East Providence, RI 02914, USA
* University Orthopedics, 1 Kettle Point Avenue, East Providence, RI 02914.
E-mail address: apcweiss@brown.edu

Hand Clin 36 (2020) 215–219
https://doi.org/10.1016/j.hcl.2020.01.012

materials of minimal value from industry. The AAOS recommends a value of less than $100.[1] This allowable cannot occur if the minor gift is for direct use of industry products. The best policy for hand surgeons is to only accept very minor gifts in random situations in no way related to direct clinical care. An example might be accepting a beer after a day at a medical convention or a medical publication of interest to the physician. Physicians must have the patients' best interests in mind in any industry dealings and need to be careful if they are in a position to influence the use of a particular product within their institutions.

If a physician recommends or can influence the use of a specific product or service provided by industry and has a financial or other personal interest in that product or service, disclosure is mandatory. This type of disclosure should be to the institution and the patient. Physicians must disclose to their institutions if they propose using a specific product or service and have any type of interest in that product or service. Importantly, the same principle applies to patients. One fairly straightforward method of accomplishing this is to provide all new patients with a written disclosure of all such conflicts of interest that the physician may hold on initial check-in for their clinical appointment. In addition, if a physician has a financial interest in an industry product and that product is used by that physician or any other physicians within their sphere of influence (eg, their institution, university, or hospital), the physician should receive no financial proceeds from that product's use (eg, royalty payment).

Consulting agreements between physicians and industry also need careful management. Any consulting performed by physicians must be by a written agreement and there should be proof of services being performed by the physician to justify any financial compensation. In addition, physicians may only receive fair market value payments, and any payments cannot be based on the value or volume of clinical efforts by the physician using that company's products or services.

Physicians should not receive any financial support from industry for any activity that does not have educational value (eg, social event). If physicians attend a Continuing Medical Education (CME) event, they should not receive any financial assistance to attend that event unless they are faculty actively teaching at the event. Physicians who present clinical results or laboratory research on products in which they have a financial interest need to disclose the conflict of interest during the presentation and only report unbiased, truthful findings.

DEALING WITH INDUSTRY FOR THE SURGEON INVENTOR

Nearly all hand surgeons, at some point in their careers, think of an idea or process to accomplish a specific surgical procedure better or faster or more predictably. If there is an interest and market to potentially turn this idea into an actionable product, then a careful understanding of the advantages and pitfalls of developing such a product is essential. There are 2 basic ways to approach product development. The first method is to go it alone. The advantages of this approach are the ability to keep the development secret, to reap a larger reward when commercialization does occur, and to control the entire process. The disadvantages include the lack of infrastructure for development and lower financial resources available compared with industry, the generally greater development time required by so-called bootstrapping the product, and the overall greater risk of failure. The second method is to approach industry early and negotiate a codevelopment process. There are several essential steps to this path. In general order, these include:

1. Documenting your idea (prepatent). The more detail you can provide an industry partner, the more likely that they will express interest. Drawings or detailed written paperwork is important. It may be best to notarize these before any meeting to establish your idea's date of creation. If you just present an oral idea, do not be surprised if you garner little interest from companies. In addition, your idea has to be practical and cannot involve something for which the technology does not exist or is overly costly.

2. Approaching a company to obtain a meeting is easier than might be imagined. The director of product development or business development is the ideal person to approach. This approach is generally easier in smaller companies (fewer roadblocks and easier to identify the correct person) but can be achieved even with the largest medical device firms. The Web sites generally identify the correct individual. Alternatively, a company representative who you know from the operating room can usually get the correct person's contact information. An introduction e-mail is usually enough. Do not provide too much information. Introduce yourself and the general topic or principle that your idea solves. Any market size information that you can research and provide is also helpful. Do not provide too much information before a meeting in person; just try to get the company interested enough to set up a meeting. A

common approach is to meet at one of several upcoming national meetings so that your travel is already preplanned. A company may be intrigued enough that they will travel directly to you to see what you have in detail; this is more common if you have a history of successful product development.

3. Sign a nondisclosure agreement (NDA) before disclosing any details of your idea. Most companies have standard form NDAs. Be sure to read it. The NDA should say that both parties agree to keep disclosed information confidential. Remember that, in the United States, the patent process is first to file, meaning that the entity that files a patent first (as opposed to the entity that first invents) is generally awarded the patent. So disclosure needs to be done with care. The patent process can be expensive and complicated, so using company funds, as opposed to your funds, has a significant advantage.

4. Negotiating an agreement requires understanding the process and desired outcome. Basic negotiating skills can be learned by anybody and encompass many parts to achieve the final result. Although the topic of negotiation is complex, a summary has been published in The Journal of Hand Surgery.[2] There are a series of basic steps and parameters to be covered (Table 1).

5. The type of agreement between an inventor and a company may vary. If the inventors have used their own resources or the resources of a small group of investors to fund the invention, and have applied for and received a patent, they are in a stronger negotiating position than if the invention is simply in the idea phase. Likewise, if the inventors have received US Food and Drug Administration (FDA) clearance for marketing, they are in the strongest possible position to achieve a strong result. The general outcomes that might be expected are highlighted in Table 2.

6. The codevelopment process requires a substantial investment of time on the inventor's part. The inventor must be prepared to work closely with the company's engineering and marketing staff during the process. In addition, if FDA clearance is required, time preparing for the eventual submission can be substantial. Often, this investment of time is not compensated and is considered part of the overall agreement.

WHAT CAN YOU EXPECT FROM DEVELOPMENT WITH INDUSTRY?

Aside from starting your own company, which is beyond the scope of this article, the eventual relationship with codeveloping an invention with industry can be rewarding by helping advance medical treatment and patient outcomes, getting a sense of accomplishment in achieving your goals, and achieving a financial return for your extensive efforts. If you can get an equity stake in a smaller company and the company eventually gets acquired by a larger strategic firm, the financial returns can be outsized. More commonly, the inventor gets a royalty-based agreement that pays quarterly, while the patent is enforceable, which can be very

Table 1
Steps of negotiation

	Definition	Subsidiary Considerations
Term	The period of time over which the license will extend	• When will it start? • When will it end? • Can it be renewed?
Exclusivity	The extent of the licensor's rights to license the IP to other parties	• Exclusivity favors the licensee • Nonexclusivity favors the licensor
Advance	Amount to be paid by the licensee at the start of the licensing period	• What is the amount? • Is it against royalties? • Or in addition to royalties?
Royalty	Recurring percentage of net sales to be paid by the licensee during the licensing period	• What is the percentage? • Will it change with time? • How often will licensee pay?
Assignability	The extent of the licensee's rights to transfer the license to other parties	• Is the license transferable? • Transferability favors the licensee • Must licensor approve? • Approval favors the licensor

Abbreviation: IP, intellectual property.

From Eltorai A, Zdeblick TA, Weiss APC. Orthopaedic Technology Innovation: A Step-by-Step Guide from Concept to Commercialization. Philadelphia: Wolters Kluwer; 2020; with permission.

Table 2
Outcome expectations from varying stages of development

Status of Invention	Likely Outcomes of Negotiation
Finished design, patent and FDA cleared	Sale of invention, licensing agreement and/or equity stake, start-up
Finished design and patent	Licensing agreement and/or equity stake, start-up, consulting
Finished design	Licensing (royalty agreement), start-up, consulting
Idea phase of invention	Licensing (royalty agreement)

Some of the likely outcomes depend on the status of the company with which you are negotiating. With larger, established companies, the outcome is most frequently royalty agreements alone based on sales revenues ± consulting agreement. With smaller or start-up companies, it may be possible to negotiate equity stake (stock grants or stock options), a consulting-based or royalty-based agreement, or both. Some of your outcome will depend on the market size of your idea, your own reputation, and the degree of the company's interest in your invention.

rewarding over time. Industry royalties vary depending on many factors but generally range from 2% to 6% of net sales of the product. Of course, if your invention does not sell well, then your work will have little financial return on your investment of time and effort. The entire process is always one of risk/return calculation for both the inventor and the company. The inventor always has to remember that companies need to risk substantial amounts of capital and employee time and effort to bring your idea to an end point. The entire process is a balancing act among all involved.[3]

Another point to consider is that, if your invention is very popular with good clinical outcomes, it will almost certainly be copied by other firms, regardless of the patent status, by engineering around the patent. The costs of filing infringement legal claims are extremely high so, if your product does not have substantial revenues, the costs outweigh the benefits, even for very large, financially sound companies. This event has happened to me several times and I view it as a confirmation of my ideas rather than from a financial loss perspective. In the end, doing something good for patient outcomes outweighs most other considerations.

In addition, what are the tax implications of your financial return for your invention? Although the rules

are constantly changing and will likely change even more in the future, these implications can be significant. Long-term versus short-term (holding period of equity for 1 year or greater in the former case) capital gains can have a profound effect on overall return. In the case of equity, filing an 83b election with the Internal Revenue Service (IRS) for stock issued that still has a low value can be advantageous long term.[4] Stock options are not stock shares. They are the option to purchase shares at a set price (determined at the time of an option grant) within a fixed period of time (commonly 5 years but this can vary). Obviously, if you exercise the options when the shares are still worth the option grant value, you are gaining nothing in value and therefore owe no tax on any gain. If you wait and the company shares increase in value, your options also become more valuable so, when exercised, you will owe tax on the difference in value between the share value at the time of exercise and the share value of the option when it was issued. Therefore, if you believe in the company's future at the time of the option grant, it is often useful to exercise the options immediately (yes, you will have to pay for those shares at the time of exercising them) because, when the shares become more valuable over time, you are not taxed until you sell the shares. In contrast, you can simply hold the shares until just before their expiration date, exercise the option grant, then pay the tax due, but you may have to wait for those shares to be valued. This method allows you to see how the company is truly doing over time before committing any money of your own.

Royalties, although reported separately from classic income, are taxed in the year they are received just like income. In certain circumstances, it is possible to write off expenses of development and other costs against this royalty income, but the rules are strict. You should consider setting up a separate limited liability company (LLC) for your projects outside normal work as the ability to write off the costs of activities directly related to these activities, which may reduce your overall tax burden of income received. The more you can convince the IRS that you are actively involved in the activities, the less they will view any such activities as passive (which can have a higher tax burden). Of course, tax advice should only come from your tax representatives and depends on the laws at the time at issue. The information presented here is for a general guide and should not be construed as tax advice.

SUMMARY

The relationship between surgeons and industry can be rewarding on multiple fronts. However, care must be taken to manage the relationship.

Whether or not your involvement is passive (involves a product in which you have no conflict of interest) or active (you have a conflict of interest in the product) influences the dynamic. One way to view this potential issue is to look at your situation with an outsider's eye. How would someone who knew all your dealings with industry react to your actions? If you know that that someone would look unfavorably on your actions, it is best to reassess them. Of course, success frequently breeds envy in others, so you have to separate that possibility out of the assessment.

DISCLOSURE

The author has nothing to disclose.

REFERENCES

1. American Academy of Orthopaedic Surgeons. Standards of professionalism, orthopaedist-industry conflicts of interest. Rosemont (IL): AAOS; 2007.

2. Weiss APC. Negotiation: how to be effective. J Hand Surg 2017;42:53–6.

3. Ragan SM. Chapter 19: Alternative pathways: Reconsidering licensing and/or co-development. In: Eltorai AEM, Zdeblick TA, Weiss APC, editors. Orthopaedic technology innovation. The Netherlands: Wolters Kluwer, Alphen aan den Rijn; 2020. p. 292–303.

4. Available at: https://www.irs.gov/pub/irs-drop/rp-12-29.pdf. Accessed June 25, 2012.

Establishment of a National Hand Surgery Data Registry
An Avenue for Quality Improvement

Robert L. Kane, BS[a], Jacob S. Nasser, BS[b], Kevin C. Chung, MD, MS[c],*

KEYWORDS

• National registry • Clinical registry • Outcomes • Quality improvement • Value

KEY POINTS

• As the health care system in the United States transitions to a value-based system, there is an increasing demand for subspecialty surgical leaders to facilitate transparency of outcomes, provide national benchmarks, and engage clinicians in a culture of quality improvement.
• Clinical registries have gained international recognition for their ability to reduce variation in practice, improve quality of care, and control cost.
• A registry for hand surgery can be an important tool for developing and tracking quality measures that are specific to the ambulatory and discretionary nature of hand surgery.

INTRODUCTION

The United States spent approximately $3.5 trillion on health care in 2017, which equates to 18% of its Gross Domestic Product.[1] Despite this extraordinary expenditure, patient outcomes in the United States rank lower than other developed nations that are spending far less per capita.[2] Health policy makers aim to reverse this trend by incentivizing a value-based model of health care delivery, where high-quality care is provided at the lowest cost.[3] Intensive efforts are underway to reduce wasteful spending and find new opportunities for quality improvement.[4,5] Variation in clinical practice has been identified as an important cause of low-value care in numerous surgical specialties.[6–9] For example, substantial regional variation exists for length of stay and cost associated with autologous free flap breast reconstruction in the United States.[9] Patients in western states stayed in the hospital significantly longer and consumed more resources, despite achieving similar outcomes to patients on the east coast.[9] A key contributor to unwarranted variations in care is the physician's own attitudes and biases toward specific treatments and diagnostics.[10,11] Therefore, reducing variation at the provider level represents an important avenue to improve quality and reduce health care spending.

Variation in clinical practice has been increasingly investigated in hand surgery. Comparative effectiveness research shows promise for reducing variations in care by giving clinicians a scientific basis for choosing one treatment over another.[12] However, translating evidence into daily practice has proved challenging. For example, studies show that simple complete trapeziectomy has comparable effectiveness and lower cost to ligament arthroplasty techniques.[13,14] Nonetheless, Yuan and colleagues[13] found that hand surgeons in Florida overwhelmingly choose trapeziectomy with ligament arthroplasty for treatment of basilar thumb arthritis. A survey of more than 800 surgeons from the American Society for Surgery of the Hand

[a] Michigan Center for Hand Outcomes and Innovation Research, 2800 Plymouth Road, Building 14, Suite G200, Ann Arbor, MI 48109, USA; [b] George Washington School of Medicine and Health Sciences, Washington, DC, USA; [c] Section of Plastic Surgery, University of Michigan Medical School, Ann Arbor, MI, USA
* Corresponding author. University of Michigan Comprehensive Hand Center, Michigan Medicine, 1500 East Medical Center Drive, 2130 Taubman Center, SPC 5340, Ann Arbor, MI 48109-5340.
E-mail address: kecchung@med.umich.edu

Hand Clin 36 (2020) 221–229
https://doi.org/10.1016/j.hcl.2020.01.007

corroborates these findings, with only 15% of respondents using current evidence as the basis for their choice of treatment of basilar thumb arthritis.[15] Estimates suggest that if simple trapeziectomy was the procedure of choice for US hand surgeons, Medicare services would save $74 million.[14]

Clinical registries have gained international recognition for their ability to reduce variation in practice, improve quality of care, and control cost.[16] Sweden has established more than 100 clinical registries, known there by the term "national quality registries," which function as powerful vehicles for quality improvement.[17] Clinical registries capture data in real time using a tightly standardized collection process across all participating clinical sites.[18] The result is a continuous monitoring system that accumulates a wealth of information on provider decision making and patient outcomes for a specific therapy, disease, or medical specialty.[18] Drolet and Lorenzi[19] identified 6 key features that distinguish a clinical registry from a regular database (**Fig. 1**).

Clinicians can use registries to identify variation patterns in processes of care and outcomes on a national scale. Furthermore, registries can be used to track provider adherence to treatment guidelines and ultimately pinpoint areas of practice that need improvement.[18] A major advantage of a clinical registry being used on a national scale is that an intervention's outcome can be examined under real-world conditions with broad inclusion criteria.[20] Compared with a randomized controlled trial, a national registry can draw conclusions that more faithfully represent the full spectrum of institutional settings, provider volume and experience, and patient demographic characteristics.[20]

Registries are recognized as integral to the future of value-based care, yet no registry exists for the field of hand surgery in the United States.[18] As excessive variation in hand care continues in the United States, patients receive care that is low quality and not cost-effective, features that are inconsistent with the value-based goal of our health care system and economy. A contributing factor is that many hand surgeons have no way of knowing how their treatment approach and associated patient outcomes compare with their peers.[21] This review article aims to demonstrate the potential of a national hand surgery data registry. Furthermore, we will use the experiences of previously successful health care registries to provide recommendations for the development of a hand surgery registry.

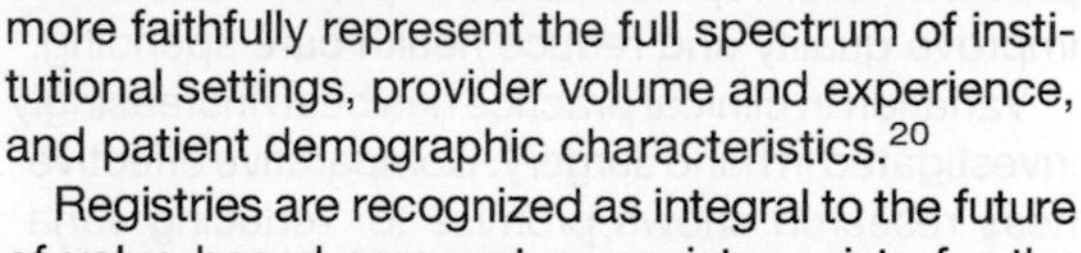

WHY DOES HAND SURGERY NEED A NATIONAL REGISTRY?

There is increasing demand for transparency of outcomes and a need for national benchmarking in hand surgery.[22] The Hand Surgery Quality Consortium has expressed their support for a national registry that tracks quality measures and improves outcomes through sharing of knowledge between hand surgeons.[22] The registry can make quality improvement a routine activity for hand surgeons and encourage them to learn from feedback on their performance. Streamlining reimbursements for providers is another important utility of registries. In the era of value-based care, pay-for-performance measures are used to determine provider reimbursements.[20] The Centers for Medicare and Medicaid Services (CMS) are using provider participation in eligible registries as a way to link quality care with reimbursement. Qualified Clinical Data Registries (QCDRs) are registries that CMS endorsed for their ability to demonstrate quality improvement. CMS incentivizes physician participation in QCDRs by permitting data submission to satisfy a component of the Quality Payment Program. A national registry for hand surgery would benefit providers by facilitating their reimbursement for quality care.

Compared with other medical specialties, quality improvement is still in early development for hand surgery, making a national registry an appealing solution.[23] Waljee and Curtin[23] identified 4 areas of quality care that are most relevant for hand surgery: outcomes, cost, safety, and patient satisfaction. A national registry can deliver an impactful and meaningful improvement to each component of this conceptual model for quality in hand care.

HOW CAN A NATIONAL REGISTRY IMPROVE OUTCOMES FOR HAND SURGERY?

In 2002, The American Society for Plastic Surgeons launched Tracking Operations and Outcomes for Plastic Surgery (TOPS), a clinical registry with QCDR status that is free for plastic surgeons.[24] TOPS has been instrumental in characterizing the

Clinical Registry

- Defined by a specific population
- Collects a predefined list of standardized data
- Collects data prospectively
- Permits comparison of aggregated data
- Requires collection of follow-up data
- Facilitates continuity of data from follow-up visits

Fig. 1. Distinguishing features of a clinical registry.

complication types and rates for plastic surgery. For example, the registry identified infection and hematoma as the most common complications for abdominoplasty and breast augmentation, respectively.[20] Risk-adjusted outcomes from plastic surgeons are aggregated and serve as benchmarks that permit providers to compare their own performance against national averages. Similarly, a national registry for hand surgery could track outcomes and develop national benchmarks not only for adverse events but also for outcomes more relevant to the field, such as health-related quality of life measures. This would give clinicians insight into their own performance and increase their awareness for potential areas of practice that need improvement.

When discussing how a registry would benefit US hand surgeons, it is important to examine what has already been done by other nations. There are currently 5 national registries that collect data on hand surgery outcomes (**Fig. 2**).[25] The first national registry made exclusively for hand surgery was HAKIR (Handkirurgiskt kvalitetsregister, Swedish for "Hand Surgery Quality Registry"), launched by the Swedish Society for Surgery of the Hand in 2010.[26] HAKIR has amassed data on over 100,000 hand operations and 70,000

questionnaires containing patient-reported outcomes (PROs). The design of this registry can serve as an important model when considering a national registry for hand surgery in the United States. In addition, a review of HAKIR's achievements provides a window into the possibilities for improving outcomes in hand care, such as using PROs to increase opportunities for shared decision making with future patients.[26]

The HAKIR development team recognized the necessity of PROs for quality improvement in hand surgery and incorporated these measures into the registry framework.[26] Patients' responses to the QuickDASH questionnaire, along with additional questions on patient satisfaction and symptoms, are recorded preoperatively and postoperatively.[26] In addition to tracking PROs, the registry records diagnosis codes, procedure codes, and complications that result in reoperation.[26] A more extensive registration process is available for surgery involving joint implants, basilar thumb arthritis, flexor tendon injury, Dupuytren contracture, and nerve injuries. For these procedures, data from preoperative and postoperative functional assessment, as well as specific surgical technique and implant model, can be tracked.[26]

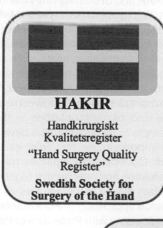

HAKIR

Handkirurgiskt
Kvalitetsregister

"Hand Surgery Quality
Register"

Swedish Society for
Surgery of the Hand

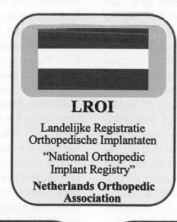

LROI

Landelijke Registratie
Orthopedische Implantaten

"National Orthopedic
Implant Registry"

Netherlands Orthopedic
Association

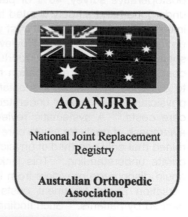

AOANJRR

National Joint Replacement
Registry

Australian Orthopedic
Association

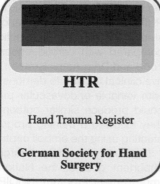

HTR

Hand Trauma Register

German Society for Hand
Surgery

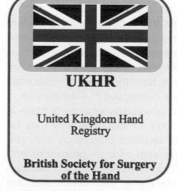

UKHR

United Kingdom Hand
Registry

British Society for Surgery
of the Hand

Fig. 2. Five national registries that collect data related to hand surgery.

Data reports from HAKIR identified the top 3 causes of reoperation for hand surgery in Sweden as postoperative infection, osteosynthesis-related complications, and joint contracture.[27] This information provides a more definitive understanding of where to focus efforts to decrease complication rates. HAKIR ultimately fosters a learning environment where providers are encouraged to share approaches that result in the best outcomes and learn from colleagues in areas where they are underperforming.[26] The registry provides regular reports that are accessible to providers and administrators. These reports have the capacity to expedite translation of evidence into practice, such as readily identifying providers who could benefit from adopting high-value treatment practices, such as simple trapeziectomy.

HOW CAN A NATIONAL REGISTRY REDUCE HEALTH CARE EXPENDITURE FOR HAND SURGERY?

Registries can drive down cost of care by improving outcomes.[28] However, they may be able to accomplish even more by tracking costs directly. For further context, consider the following insights from patient-provider interactions. In a postoperative survey, 48% of patients who had undergone hand surgery wanted their surgeon to initiate a conversation about cost when treatment options were presented.[29] However, only 7% of surveyed patients had the opportunity to discuss cost of care.[29] One explanation may be related to evidence that shows a substantial number of physicians have a poor understanding of health care costs.[30] A systematic review of physician awareness of costs for health care services determined that only one-third of physicians had an accurate understanding.[30] This lack of knowledge could discourage providers from initiating a conversation about treatment costs that is much desired by patients.[29] Such findings are concerning given that provider decision making has the greatest influence on health care costs.[31]

Registries present the opportunity for providers to directly track resource usage and estimated costs incurred from care.[32] This can increase transparency of provider-level health care expenditure and show providers how their use of resources compares with their colleagues.[33] Furthermore, it is conceivable that physicians who participate in tracking costs through a national registry may be better equipped to facilitate discussion with patients regarding the cost of their procedure and follow-up care.[33] This encourages shared decision making through identifying treatments that are congruent with patient cost preferences.[34] If

providers are routinely engaged in tracking the costs associated with their decisions and can compare their own data with national benchmarks, they may feel more empowered in their role to manage the rising costs of health care.[33] Currently, the only national registry that collects data on the cost of hand procedures is The Hand Trauma Register, founded by the Germany Society of Hand Surgery.[25] A comprehensive national registry for hand surgery in the United States could be the first to collect estimated costs of care for hand procedures in real time from routine clinical practice.

HOW CAN A NATIONAL REGISTRY IMPROVE SAFETY FOR HAND SURGERY?

The first quality improvement registries were created to track implants used for arthroplasty.[35] An important goal for these registries was to detect faulty prosthetic devices before widespread use occurred.[35] The Swedish Knee Arthroplasty Register (SKAR) began collecting data in 1975 and is regarded as the first registry focused on quality improvement.[26,35] SKAR was able to track outcomes, such as revision rate, for each prosthesis based on manufacturer and model.[35] In 1979, the Swedish Hip Arthroplasty Register (SHAR) was developed.[26] The SKAR and SHAR registries identified implant models with higher-than-expected failure rates and dictated whether specific implants should be removed from the market. The results from these registries led to advancements, such as discovering that rheumatoid arthritis was a contraindication for unicompartmental knee replacement.[35] In addition, Sweden maintains one of the lowest revision rates for knee and hip arthroplasties in the world.[35,36] This example highlights medical device surveillance as an important use for registries in quality improvement. Governmental agencies have recognized this application and now require registry participation for certain device manufacturers as a condition of postmarket approval.[21,37] For instance, the Stenting and Angioplasty with Protection of Patients with High Risk for Endarterectomy (SAPPHIRE) trial showed noninferiority of carotid artery stenting with a distal embolic protection device compared with carotid endarterectomy.[38,39] The Food and Drug Administration required a prospective clinical registry to demonstrate that physicians with variable endovascular procedure experience could produce similar outcomes to SAPPHIRE if they followed a training program in carotid artery stenting using the emboli capture device.[38,39]

Measuring the safety of surgical procedures is an important goal of the National Surgical Quality Improvement Program (NSQIP), a clinical registry led by the American College of Surgeons.[28] The business model for NSQIP and many other national registries rests on the fact that payment for participation will supply data that can be used by clinicians to drive down complication rates and wasted resources, achieving overall net savings.[28] NSQIP contains the largest quantity of risk-adjusted surgical outcome data in the United States.[28] Variables, such as mortality rates, complication rates, and length of stay are collected.[28] Although this registry model works well for the field of general surgery, hand surgery is typically performed in an ambulatory setting and has minimal mortality rates.[23] In recent years, CMS has created a list of surgical safety measures that are applicable to the ambulatory setting, all of which influence reimbursement.[23] A registry designed by hand surgery leaders could take this concept one step further by identifying additional safety measures that are specific to patients with particular hand conditions.[23]

HOW CAN A NATIONAL REGISTRY IMPROVE PATIENT SATISFACTION IN HAND SURGERY?

Patient satisfaction and experience are recognized as key measurements of quality care.[40] Satisfaction and experience are often used interchangeably, but they represent distinct concepts of quality (**Fig. 3**).[41,42] Patient experience at US hospitals is measured by the CMS using a standardized survey called The Hospital Consumer Assessment of Healthcare Providers and Systems (HCAHPS).[43] CMS factors the HCAHPS score into value-based payments for hospitals and Medicare reimbursement, which highlights the major influence that patient experience has in the US health care system.[40] Although HCAHPS monitors structures and processes of care as experienced by hospitalized patients, these data do not reliably correlate with actual treatment outcomes.[44] Moreover, the survey focuses on general measures that are applicable to all inpatients and may overlook processes that are more important for hand procedures. A

national registry for hand surgery can be an initiative that reimagines how the patient's perception of care can fuel better quality measures. The registry should be designed to collect structure and processes measures that more closely reflect a high-quality patient experience that is specific to the ambulatory setting of hand surgery. The registry can also track PROs to inform clinicians on how to increase patient satisfaction. For example, HAKIR aggregated PROs to create an interactive online experience for patients who are considering surgical treatment options.[26] New patients can view average changes in pain and functionality associated with particular interventions, helping to align their expectations with available evidence and promote patient satisfaction.[26]

Asking hand surgery patients how they define quality is an important direction for research studies. Eppler and colleagues[34] performed a qualitative analysis that revealed 4 themes of high-quality hand surgery as defined by hand surgery patients themselves (**Fig. 4**). Of these 4 themes, regaining hand function with the least amount of pain was the only one that is currently measured as a mainstay of practice.[34] To facilitate tracking the other aspects of care that hand patients value, a registry may offer a solution. The registry can track standardized process measures, such as offering multiple educational materials, discussing out-of-pocket cost of treatment, and assessing potential psychosocial barriers that could impact recovery and outcomes. To make this more feasible, data collection could be performed by providers and ancillary staff so that these conversations occur with those most qualified to facilitate the proper discussion.

DESIGNING AND FUNDING THE REGISTRY

Planning the registry begins with identifying a specific purpose and associated patient population for investigation. The objective must coincide

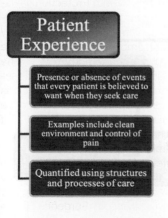
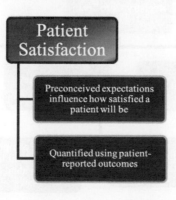

Fig. 3. Comparing patient satisfaction with patient experience.

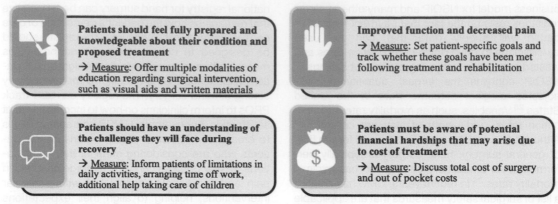

Patients should feel fully prepared and knowledgeable about their condition and proposed treatment
→ Measure: Offer multiple modalities of education regarding surgical intervention, such as visual aids and written materials

Improved function and decreased pain
→ Measure: Set patient-specific goals and track whether these goals have been met following treatment and rehabilitation

Patients should have an understanding of the challenges they will face during recovery
→ Measure: Inform patients of limitations in daily activities, arranging time off work, additional help taking care of children

Patients must be aware of potential financial hardships that may arise due to cost of treatment
→ Measure: Discuss total cost of surgery and out of pocket costs

Fig. 4. Quality of care measures defined by hand surgery patients.

with questions that the registry aims to answer for the field of hand surgery.[45] Examples could be investigating provider-level variation patterns in outcomes of common hand interventions, surveilling prosthetic devices and implants for the fingers and wrist, or further defining the epidemiology of hand conditions. In addition, choosing a well-defined goal for the registry permits identification of potential stakeholders who would want to assume critical roles in the next steps in development.[32] Next, a steering or executive committee must be selected to oversee the design and operation of all major divisions within the registry.[45] To build a registry with a national scope, the steering committee must also assemble experts across a diverse set of disciplines who make up the core registry team (**Fig. 5**).[32] A key decision for the steering committee is to define the specific data elements that the registry will collect.[45] The HAKIR developers recommend starting the registry with a few data elements that are simple to collect.[26] In addition, regularly eliciting feedback from staff members who

perform data collection can identify opportunities to improve the collection routine.

Securing adequate financial support is arguably the greatest challenge that the steering committee will face.[45] The stakeholders should be aware that the greater the scope and patient volume of the registry, the costlier the operations become. A key motivation for investors is access and use of the registry data. Therefore, it is important to recognize which organizations and stakeholders have the most to gain from partnering with the registry, as these may be the parties most willing to invest.[46] The steering committee should develop a project plan that shows potential investors a clear timeline for deliverables and a general business model for how the registry can be sustained in the long term.[46] Financial backing from governmental health care agencies should be solicited, as these groups may provide federal grants due to their interests in conducting comparative effectiveness research and promoting value-based care. Medical professional societies, device manufacturers, and nonprofit disease foundations are

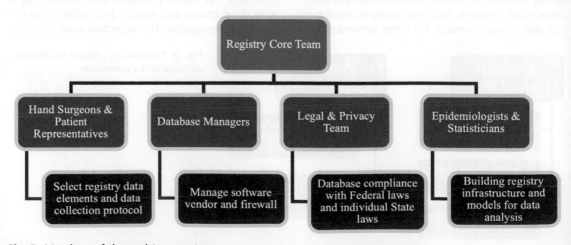

Fig. 5. Members of the registry core team.

also important avenues for financial support.[32] Finally, registries may generate revenue through membership fees from individual providers or institutions. These fees can be designed in multiple tiers so that the registry can charge more money by providing greater access to data or more in-depth analytical reports.[47] The business model must plan ahead to secure funding sources both for startup and for maintaining operations in the long run.[47]

The long-term benefits of registries are capable of substantial positive returns on investment.[28,48] The Australian Commission on Safety and Quality in Health Care performed a cost-effectiveness analysis for 5 prominent Australian clinical quality registries.[48] The study converted registry-derived improvements in outcomes and resource use into economic value, then measured these data against the costs required to launch and maintain these registries.[48] The results showed that since their launch date, all 5 registries had a positive return on investment costs.[48] Further economic analysis has been performed by The Boston Consulting Group (BCG).[49] In 2009, the BCG was hired by Swedish health care leaders to investigate expansion of the nation's clinical registries.[50] The BCG found that an investment of $70 million in Swedish registries each year could decrease annual growth in health care expenditures from 4.7% to 4.1%, which equated to a $7 billion reduction in costs over a period of 10 years.[50] Furthermore, the BCG analyzed hip arthroplasty revision rates between the United States and Sweden, and determined that Sweden avoided 7500 revisions for arthroplasty between 2000 and 2009 by maintaining a lower revision rate relative to that of the United States.[50] By comparison, if the United States had achieved the same revision rate as Sweden, it could have avoided $2 billion spent on revision care between 2005 and 2015.[50]

SUMMARY

Surgical registries offer a seemingly endless number of possibilities for improving quality, lowering costs, and increasing shared decision making with patients. In addition, a hand surgery registry can serve as an important tool for developing and tracking quality measures that are specific to the ambulatory and often discretionary nature of hand surgery. Design of the registry will require diverse stakeholders with a strong interest in the registry's data, as well as a clear plan to solicit proper financial support. The best approach for implementing a registry is to begin with a well-defined goal, collect a few basic variables, and then repeatedly refine the data collection routine.

Once this critical foundation has been solidified, the registry can slowly expand to reach national coverage, along with tracking more complex variables, such as PROs.

FINANCIAL DISCLOSURE

Dr K.C. Chung receives funding from the National Institutes of Health and book royalties from Wolters Kluwer and Elsevier.

CONFLICTS OF INTEREST

The authors have no conflicts of interest to report.

REFERENCES

1. Centers for Medicare and Medicaid Services. National health expenditure data. 2018. Available at: https://www.cms.gov/Research-Statistics-Data-and-Systems/Statistics-Trends-and-Reports/NationalHealthExpendData/NationalHealthAccountsHistorical.html. Accessed September 29, 2019.
2. Papanicolas I, Woskie LR, Jha AK. Health care spending in the United States and other high-income countries. JAMA 2018;319(10):1024–39.
3. Srinivasan D, Desai NR. The impact of the transition from volume to value on heart failure care: implications of novel payment models and quality improvement initiatives. J Card Fail 2017;23(8):615–20.
4. Burwell SM. Setting value-based payment goals—HHS efforts to improve U.S. health care. N Engl J Med 2015;372(10):897–9.
5. Fleurence R, Whicher D, Dunham K, et al. The patient-centered outcomes research institute's role in advancing methods for patient-centered outcomes research. Med Care 2015;53(1):2–8.
6. Urbach DR, Baxter NN. Reducing variation in surgical care. BMJ 2005;330(7505):1401–2.
7. Ugiliweneza B, Kong M, Nosova K, et al. Spinal surgery: variations in health care costs and implications for episode-based bundled payments. Spine (Phila Pa 1976) 2014;39(15):1235–42.
8. Ayanian JZ, Guadagnoli E. Variations in breast cancer treatment by patient and provider characteristics. Breast Cancer Res Treat 1996;40(1):65–74.
9. Billig JI, Lu Y, Momoh AO, et al. A nationwide analysis of cost variation for autologous free flap breast reconstruction. JAMA Surg 2017;152(11):1039–47.
10. Birkmeyer JD, Reames BN, McCulloch P, et al. Understanding of regional variation in the use of surgery. Lancet 2013;382(9898):1121–9.
11. Becker SJ, Teunis T, Blauth J, et al. Medical services and associated costs vary widely among surgeons treating patients with hand osteoarthritis. Clin Orthop Relat Res 2015;473(3):1111–7.

12. Johnson SP, Chung KC. Comparative effectiveness research in hand surgery. Hand Clin 2014;30(3): 319–27, vi.

13. Yuan F, Aliu O, Chung KC, et al. Evidence-based practice in the surgical treatment of thumb carpometacarpal joint arthritis. J Hand Surg Am 2017; 42(2):104–12.e1.

14. Mahmoudi E, Yuan F, Lark ME, et al. Medicare spending and evidence-based approach in surgical treatment of thumb carpometacarpal joint arthritis: 2001 to 2010. Plast Reconstr Surg 2016;137(6): 980e–9e.

15. Deutch Z, Niedermeier SR, Awan HM. Surgeon preference, influence, and treatment of thumb carpometacarpal arthritis. Hand (N Y) 2018;13(4):403–11.

16. Larsson S, Lawyer P, Garellick G, et al. Use of 13 disease registries in 5 countries demonstrates the potential to use outcome data to improve health care's value. Health Aff (Millwood) 2012;31(1):220–7.

17. Nilsson E, Orwelius L, Kristenson M. Patient-reported outcomes in the Swedish National Quality Registers. J Intern Med 2016;279(2):141–53.

18. Bhatt DL, Drozda JP Jr, Shahian DM, et al. ACC/AHA/STS statement on the future of registries and the performance measurement enterprise: a report of the American College of Cardiology/American Heart Association Task Force on Performance Measures and The Society of Thoracic Surgeons. J Am Coll Cardiol 2015;66(20):2230–45.

19. Drolet BC, Lorenzi NM. Registries and evidence-based medicine in craniofacial and plastic surgery. J Craniofac Surg 2012;23(1):301–3.

20. Alderman AK, Collins ED, Streu R, et al. Benchmarking outcomes in plastic surgery: national complication rates for abdominoplasty and breast augmentation. Plast Reconstr Surg 2009;124(6): 2127–33.

21. Hume KM, Crotty CA, Simmons CJ, et al. Medical specialty society-sponsored data registries: opportunities in plastic surgery. Plast Reconstr Surg 2013;132(1):159e–67e.

22. Kamal RN, Kakar S, Ruch D, et al. Quality measurement: a primer for hand surgeons. J Hand Surg Am 2016;41(5):645–51.

23. Waljee JF, Curtin C. Quality assessment in hand surgery. Hand Clin 2014;30(3):329–34, vi.

24. Sinno H, Dionisopoulos T, Slavin SA, et al. The utility of outcome studies in plastic surgery. Plast Reconstr Surg Glob Open 2014;2(7):e189.

25. Vakalopoulos KA, Arner M, Denissen GAW, et al. A review of national hand surgery registries. 2019. Available at: https://hakir.se/wp-content/uploads/2019/06/Poster-ISAR-2019-9-May.pdf. Accessed September 21, 2019.

26. Arner M. Developing a national quality registry for hand surgery: challenges and opportunities. EFORT Open Rev 2016;1(4):100–6.

27. Arner M, Bartonek F, Lindblad N. HAKIR annual report 2014. 2015. Available at: https://hakir.se/wp-content/uploads/2016/04/%c3%85rsrapport_2014_LR_ENG2-MA-160324_new_up1.pdf. Accessed September 20, 2019.

28. Maggard-Gibbons M. The use of report cards and outcome measurements to improve the safety of surgical care: the American College of Surgeons National Surgical Quality Improvement Program. BMJ Qual Saf 2014;23(7):589–99.

29. Alokozai A, Crijns TJ, Janssen SJ, et al. Cost in hand surgery: the patient perspective. J Hand Surg Am 2019;44(11):992.e1-26.

30. Allan GM, Lexchin J. Physician awareness of diagnostic and nondrug therapeutic costs: a systematic review. Int J Technol Assess Health Care 2008; 24(2):158–65.

31. Crosson FJ. Change the microenvironment. Delivery system reform essential to control costs. Mod Healthc 2009;39(17):20–1.

32. Gliklich RE, Dreyer NA, Leavy MB. Registries for evaluating patient outcomes: a user's guide. Rockville (MD): Agency for Healthcare Research and Quality; 2014.

33. Sharp J. Registries in accountable care: addendum to registries for evaluating patient outcomes: a user's guide. 3rd edition. Rockville (MD): Agency for Healthcare Research and Quality; 2018.

34. Eppler SL, Kakar S, Sheikholeslami N, et al. Defining quality in hand surgery from the patient's perspective: a qualitative analysis. J Hand Surg Am 2019; 44(4):311–20.e4.

35. Robertsson O, Ranstam J, Sundberg M, et al. The Swedish knee arthroplasty register: a review. Bone Joint Res 2014;3(7):217–22.

36. Paxton EW, Cafri G, Nemes S, et al. An international comparison of THA patients, implants, techniques, and survivorship in Sweden, Australia, and the United States. Acta Orthop 2019;90(2):148–52.

37. Trotter JP. Patient registries: a new gold standard for "real world" research. Ochsner J 2002;4(4):211–4.

38. Katzen BT, Criado FJ, Ramee SR, et al. Carotid artery stenting with emboli protection surveillance study: thirty-day results of the CASES-PMS study. Catheter Cardiovasc Interv 2007;70(2):316–23.

39. Schreiber TL, Strickman N, Davis T, et al. Carotid artery stenting with emboli protection surveillance study: outcomes at 1 year. J Am Coll Cardiol 2010; 56(1):49–57.

40. Kennedy GD, Tevis SE, Kent KC. Is there a relationship between patient satisfaction and favorable outcomes? Ann Surg 2014;260(4):592–8 [discussion: 598–600].

41. Agency of Healthcare Research and Quality. What is patient experience?. 2017. Available at: https://www.ahrq.gov/cahps/about-cahps/patient-experience/index.html. Accessed September 24, 2019.

42. Al-Abri R, Al-Balushi A. Patient satisfaction survey as a tool towards quality improvement. Oman Med J 2014;29(1):3–7.

43. Centers for Medicare and Medicaid Services. HCAHPS: patients' perspectives of care survey. 2017. Available at: https://www.cms.gov/Medicare/Quality-Initiatives-Patient-Assessment-Instruments/HospitalQualityInits/HospitalHCAHPS.html. Accessed September 24, 2019.

44. Schmocker RK, Cherney Stafford LM, Winslow ER. Satisfaction with surgeon care as measured by the Surgery-CAHPS survey is not related to NSQIP outcomes. Surgery 2019;165(3):510–5.

45. Mandavia R, Knight A, Phillips J, et al. What are the essential features of a successful surgical registry? a systematic review. BMJ Open 2017;7(9):e017373.

46. National Quality Registry Network. Frequently asked questions about clinical data registries. The PCPI Foundation. 2016. Available at: https://cdn.ymaws.com/www.thepcpi.org/resource/resmgr/nqrn-clinical-registry-faq.pdf. Accessed September 24, 2019.

47. National Quality Registry Network. Clinical registry business case tool PCPI foundation. 2016. Available at: https://cdn.ymaws.com/www.thepcpi.org/resource/resmgr/nqrn-registry-business-case-.pdf. Accessed September 24, 2019.

48. Australian Commission on Safety and Quality in Healthcare. Economic evaluation of clinical quality registries. 2016. Available at: https://www.safetyandquality.gov.au/sites/default/files/migrated/Economic-evaluation-of-clinical-quality-registries-Final-report-Nov-2016.pdf. Accessed September 20, 2019.

49. The Boston Consulting Group. Value guided healthcare as a platform for industrial development in Sweden—feasibility study. 2009. Available at: https://www.bcg.com/documents/file148780.pdf. Accessed September 19, 2019.

50. Larsson S, Lawyer P. Improving health care value: the case for disease registries. The Boston Consulting Group. 2011. Available at: https://www.bcg.com/publications/2011/health-care-payers-providers-public-sector-value-based-health-care-interactive.aspx. Accessed September 20, 2019.

Deriving Evidence from Secondary Data in Hand Surgery
Strengths, Limitations, and Future Directions

Lee Squitieri, MD, PhD, MS[a],*, Kevin C. Chung, MD, MS[b]

KEYWORDS

- Registry • Hand surgery • Administrative • Claims • Electronic health records • Big data
- Secondary data analysis

KEY POINTS

- The number of secondary data sets available for health services research is rapidly increasing, but most do not include essential information required to perform impactful research in hand surgery.
- Claims data, administrative data sets, patient/disease registries, quality-improvement registries, electronic health records, and health surveys represent distinct categories of secondary data with unique strengths and limitations that are critical to understand when determining data set appropriateness for a specific study question.
- A strong foundation in statistical methods is needed to accurately link data sets and capture the full range of clinical settings and perioperative services used by hand surgery patients.
- Establishing quality collaborative initiatives and specialty-specific registries in hand surgery will allow researchers to capture detailed patient information, set benchmarks, and identify areas for quality improvement.
- Hand surgery health services researchers should engage policymakers and stakeholders early in the study design process to maximize potential impact of research results and effect changes that best serve the unique needs of the patient population.

The US health care system currently is experiencing profound change driven by rapid advancements in health information technology and increasing pressure to improve value through evidence-based health policy.[1,2] Over the past decade, the number of secondary data sets available for health services research has increased dramatically and expanded the ability to inform quality/performance measure development, payment reform, and health policy.[3–14] The large and diverse sampling pool of many secondary data sets promotes researchers to test population-based hypotheses that are otherwise too expensive or impractical to study via primary data collection. These population studies include national practice trends, geographic variation, access/outcome disparities, and cost/value of care.[11–16] Because secondary data are not collected for the purpose of evaluating specific study aims, researchers must have a strong understanding of data set construction, rigorous study design, and statistical methods to derive accurate and impactful conclusions.[17–20]

Detailed descriptions of many commonly used data sets and guidelines for statistical analysis have been published previously and should be

a Division of Plastic and Reconstructive Surgery, Department of Surgery, Keck School of Medicine, University of Southern California, 1500 San Pablo Street, Suite 415, Los Angeles, CA 90033, USA; b Division of Plastic and Reconstructive Surgery, Department of Surgery, Michigan Medicine, University of Michigan Medical School, 1500 East Medical Center Drive, 2130 Taubman Center, SPC 5340, Ann Arbor, MI 48109-5340, USA
* Corresponding author.
E-mail address: lee.squitieri@gmail.com

Hand Clin 36 (2020) 231–243
https://doi.org/10.1016/j.hcl.2020.01.011

referenced prior to performing secondary data research.[11–30] A focused discussion on the relevance and limitations of these data sets in hand surgery, however, is lacking in the current literature. Hand surgery is a very different subspecialty of surgery with distinct preoperative considerations, physical examination findings, postoperative care, and provider/organizational factors that lend themselves to unique data requirements and analytical challenges compared with other surgical fields. Furthermore, the scope of hand surgery practice across a variety of clinical settings (eg, inpatient, outpatient, and office-based) and payers (pediatrics, uninsured trauma patients, workers' compensation, employer-based, Medicare, health maintenance organizations, and so forth) deserves special attention when choosing appropriate data sources and assessing the impact of potential study conclusions.

As the number of available secondary data sets continues to expand, health services researchers in all fields must become comfortable evaluating new data sources and discriminating between various data sets for specific study questions. This article describes categories of secondary data and provides guidance on how to evaluate the appropriateness of data sources for deriving evidence in hand surgery. Issues and limitations of studying hand surgery with currently available data sets are discussed and recommendations for future research suggested.

CATEGORIES OF SECONDARY DATA

The most important part of any secondary data analysis is choosing the right data set and managing data limitations with respect to the specific research question being tested. Researchers must understand how and why the data were collected as well as the specific characteristics of each data variable in order to estimate bias, anticipate the need to link additional data sources, and determine appropriate statistical methods for analysis. As new data sets continue to emerge, it is essential to appreciate the general principles of various secondary data categories to determine whether a specific data set is appropriate to use alone or in concert with other data sources. **Table 1** provides an overview of various data categories, their strengths and limitations, and current examples within each category.

Claims Data

Claims-based data sets include individual claims for each type of financial interaction within the health care system (inpatient hospital, outpatient facilities, physician/provider, home health,

pharmacy, laboratory, therapy, durable medical equipment purchases, and so forth).[5,13,21,22] In their original form, claims are an extremely rich and comprehensive source of utilization and expenditure data but require special data safety agreements to obtain identifiable patient information that is necessary to aggregate and link claims.[5,13,21,22] For example, a hand surgery researcher wanting to study outpatient surgery requiring postoperative splints and therapy would have to acquire provider claims for the physician and therapist, facility claims for the site of surgery, durable medical equipment claims for any equipment, and any other relevant diagnostic, laboratory, or home health claims. Each claim has its own unique set of variables that must be uniformly recoded prior to aggregation or linkage at the patient or encounter level (ie, 1 row of data per patient or encounter) for meaningful analysis.[5,30]

Although labor and resource intensive, researchers using raw claims have the freedom to choose and format a variety information that is generally unavailable in other data categories, such as physical/occupational therapy visit information, equipment use, payment data, and current procedural terminology (CPT) codes.[5,16] Identifiable raw claims also contain various provider and patient information that allows longitudinal follow-up across clinical settings and linkage to other sources of useful data containing hospital characteristics and socioeconomic factors.[5] This data flexibility is incredibly useful for analyses in hand surgery for a variety of reasons. First, many hand surgery procedures occur in both inpatient and outpatient facilities and, therefore, may not be captured in administrative data sets restricted to a single clinical setting. Second, the ability to follow patients longitudinally across settings and obtain data about ancillary services (eg, physical/occupation therapy, home health, and durable medical equipment) confers substantial benefit compared with other data sources. Third, the inclusion of payment data, rather than billed charges contained in most other forms of data, is useful for studies assessing cost of care.[16] And, finally, the potential to link data to various other sources of patient and provider information makes these data compatible with a wider variety of research questions compared with other data sets.

Claims data, however, have substantial limitations. Researchers must remember that claims data are collected for the purpose of billing and coding and are not as clinically comprehensive or accurate as information in the patient medical record.[31,32] It is important to anticipate and understand potential billing/coding biases in the context of payment incentives/penalties and evaluate

Table 1
Strengths and limitations of secondary data sources in hand surgery

Data Category	Characteristics	Examples	Strengths	Weaknesses
Claims Data	Billable interactions between insured patients and the health care delivery system	• Medicare or other insurance claims • Independent analytic companies (MarketScan, PearlDiver)	• Contain detailed procedure information (CPT) • Payment (not charge) data • Variety of clinical services settings and settings of care • May link longitudinally	• Expensive • Difficult to obtain • Labor-intensive sophisticated programming required to aggregate/link patient identifiable data
Administrative Datasets	Encounter level data collected by government agencies or large health organizations	• Healthcare Cost and Utilization Project (HCUP) • California Office of Statewide Health Planning and Development (OSHPD)	• Inexpensive, easy to access • All-payer • User-friendly with a variety of analytic tools (sampling weights, cost/charge ratios) • Easily linked with other data sources • Ambulatory surgery dataset contains CPT codes	• Organized by type of encounter (not cross-setting) • Most are unable to be linked longitudinally • Charge (not payment) data
Electronic Health Records	Data obtained at the point of care at a hospital or other health care facility	• Kaiser • University health systems • Department of Veterans Affairs • County health system	• Detailed clinical and procedure information • Detailed provider/encounter data	• Traditionally confined to single health system • Machine learning techniques not well established • Does not include payment/charge data to evaluate cost

(continued on next page)

Table 1
(continued)

Data Category	Characteristics	Examples	Strengths	Weaknesses
Health Surveys	Data collected by government or other agency that combines medical information with survey data collected directly from patients	• National Health Interview Survey (NHIS) • Consumer Assessment of Healthcare Providers and Systems (CAHPS) • Medical Expenditure Panel Survey (MEPS) • National Health and Nutrition Examination Survey (NHANES) • Medicare Survey Data: https://www.cms.gov/Research-Statistics-Data-and-Systems/Research-Statistics-Data-and-Systems.html	• Inexpensive, easy to access • Contains patient-reported information that is not readily available in other forms of secondary data • Sophisticated sampling/weighting techniques • Some may be linked to other Medicare research identifiable files (RIFs)	• Limited medical/surgical information • Often unable to be used alone • Linkage among Medicare surveys can be costly and difficult
Quality Improvement Registries	Often specialty specific collaborative involving an independent data collection process of clinical information that may be later used for benchmarking and quality improvement	• National Surgical Quality Improvement Program (NSQIP) • American College of Surgeons (ACS) Quality Programs: https://www.facs.org/quality-programs • Swedish National Healthcare Quality Registry for Hand Surgery • United States Surgical Outcome System: https://surgicaloutcomesystem.com/	• Better data quality and completeness compared to administrative data or raw claims • User friendly with broader patient samples compared to single system EHR data	• Opt-in status may bias/limit sample • Labor intensive and costly process of data collection/quality assurance • Limited data collection and follow-up • No patient identifiers for direct linkage, indirect linkage requires probabilistic algorithms

| Patient or Disease Registries | Clinical information systems that track a narrow range of key data for certain medical conditions | • Surveillance Epidemiology and End Results (SEER)
• National Trauma Data Bank (NTDB)
• NIH Disease Specific Registries: https://www.nih.gov/health-information/nih-clinical-research-trials-you/list-registries
• United Kingdom National Hand Registry | • Better data quality and completeness compared to administrative data or raw claims
• User friendly with broader patient samples compared to single system EHR data
• Some may be directly linked to claims data | • Usually organized by disease or exposure, not treatment (e.g., hand surgery)
• Lack detailed information for medical conditions/procedure other than original purpose of database |

patterns of missing data, identify coding inconsistencies, and evaluate the impact of geographic diagnostic coding intensity prior to analysis.[31–37] Claims are also expensive, difficult to obtain, and require sophisticated, labor-intensive computer coding methods to aggregate or link with other appropriate data sources. In response to these limitations, several analytical companies, such as MarketScan and PearlDiver, as well as insurance payers (Blue Cross Blue Shield, Premier Health, and UnitedHealthcare) have developed ways to collaborate with researchers and create more user-friendly data constructs.[13,38,39] These data sets are also relatively expensive and require a thorough understanding of data nuances to ensure that patient sampling, variable quality, and linkage capacity are sufficient for current and future research needs.

Administrative Data

Administrative data sets are collected by governments or large health organizations for financial, quality-improvement, monitoring, or reporting purposes. The most established and widely used administrative data in the United States is the Healthcare Cost and Utilization Project (HCUP), which is overseen by the federal government under the Agency for Healthcare Research and Quality.[4,24] The HCUP family of databases contain deidentified patient information from all payers and are organized by type of encounter (inpatient, ambulatory surgery, emergency room visits, and so forth). Many of these data sets utilize a format similar to claims, but data go through additional data cleaning and quality-assurance processes to provide a more reliable and user-friendly data product.[40] Also, unlike claims data, the information contained in administrative data sets are collected directly from hospitals and providers, creating unique advantages and disadvantages for certain types of analyses.

The major benefits of administrative data are their relatively low cost, easy accessibility, and user-friendly format for most health services research.[4,20,40] For example, many of the HCUP data sets contain additional clinical information (extra diagnostic codes, provider/facility data, and so forth), facilitating linkage with other data sources, and provide a variety of analytical tools, such as sampling weights and cost-charge ratios.[4,24] Because these data utilize the same diagnosis and procedure coding as billing claims, however, they have less clinical granularity and are more prone to potential coding bias compared with data extracted directly from the medical record. Also, because administrative data are collected directly from providers/facilities, they contain charge (rather than payment) data, which may be less accurate for cost analyses.[16]

For hand surgery–specific research, there are several exciting areas of administrative data development that are important to be aware of. First, expansion of the State Ambulatory Surgery and Services Database over the past 2 decades is incredibly valuable for the field of hand surgery because these data contain CPT codes that were previously available only in claims data.[4,24] Second, increasing availability of state-level identifiable data, like the California Office of Statewide Health Planning and Development, and of HCUP supplemental files for revisit analyses now allows data to be linked at the patient level across encounters for longitudinal study in the outpatient setting.[4,8] As these new data become more robust and readily available, it is important for health services researchers in hand surgery to familiarize themselves with these resources and understand the nuanced differences in data variables across state lines and annual data revisions.

Electronic Health Records

Hospital and health system–based electronic health records (EHRs) represent the most accurate and complete source of patient health care information.[41] Data are entered directly at the point of care during patient interactions and contain detailed clinical information that are not routinely collected for billing claims, administrative data, or quality-improvement/patient registries. Traditional secondary data analyses of EHRs have been limited to single health system retrospective chart reviews. As legislation, payment policies, grant funding, and technological advancements continue to promote use and integration of EHRs across clinical settings and providers, however, these data will become a robust source of longitudinal patient information that is uniquely equipped to inform cross-setting quality of care measures, process optimization, and clinical decision-making/guidelines.[1,41,42]

Given the clinical detail required to study many questions in hand surgery (examination findings, date/mechanism of injury, and so forth), the increasing ability to apply big data techniques to EHRs is exciting and inevitably will facilitate better health services research. Hand surgery outcomes and comparative effectiveness research require unique data variables for proper risk adjustment, and harnessing this information on a large scale from EHRs will be a powerful tool in the future. Machine learning and natural language processing algorithms, however, constitute a relatively new innovation geared toward general medicine and surgery, whose specialties have language priorities and patient populations that are inherently different from those in hand surgery.[42,43] As this field grows, it will be imperative for hand surgeons to remain involved and ensure that the statistical techniques used to validate natural language processing are relevant to the unique needs of hand surgery research. Furthermore, hand surgeons involved in health services research also should be mindful of EHR data limitations and anticipate the need to link claims and/or survey data in order to study specific research questions.[44,45]

Health Surveys

Health surveys are a unique source of secondary data that combine medical information with survey data collected directly from patients. Examples include the Medical Expenditure Panel Survey, National Health Interview Survey, and Hospital Consumer Assessment of Healthcare Providers and Systems survey.[7,46,47] For health services research pertaining to quality-of-life, health attitudes/preferences, and socioeconomic determinants of health, these data sources represent a rich source of information that is not readily available in claims or administrative data, such as socioeconomic, demographic, and behavioral risk factors. Survey information is often collected over the phone by government agencies and deidentified data usually are inexpensive and relatively easy to obtain. Also, most large health surveys in the United States involve sophisticated sampling design and weighting methods so that study conclusions may be generalized on a national level.

At the present time, a majority of secondary survey data lack detailed medical information necessary for surgical research and must be linked to other data sources (eg, claims and EHRs) to conduct meaningful health services research. For example, Medicare surveys may be linked to Medicare claims data using a unique patient identifier variable.[5,32] This process, however, requires specialized data safety agreements, programming capabilities, and substantial additional cost. As the number of well-designed clinical and group survey data continues to increase and patient-reported outcome measures become widely integrated into EHRs, the availability and potential of secondary survey data in health services research surely will expand.[7,42] Refinement and availability of these data will be extremely important to augment health services research in hand surgery and facilitate assessment of practice patterns and patient-reported outcomes on a national level.[42]

Quality-Improvement Registries

Another growing source of secondary data is quality-improvement collaboratives for surgical conditions. In these models, individual providers and facilities participate in an independent data collection process of clinical information that may be used later for benchmarking and quality improvement. The most widely known surgical quality-improvement registry is the American College of Surgeons National Surgical Quality Improvement Program, which collects in-depth risk-adjusted information on 30-day surgical outcomes directly from EHRs.[3,23] By obtaining data directly from patient medical charts, these registries provide more accurate and relevant data that are less prone to coding biases than billing claims and also allow data collection for prospective clinical trials.[23,32,48] At present, these data do not provide patient identifiers for direct linkage to other data sources, but several researchers have developed indirect probabilistic algorithms to estimate linkage with claims data.[49]

The main drawback of quality-improvement registries is the labor-intensive and costly process of data collection and quality assurance. This feature often leads to mandatory participation fees and limits the ability to collect a wide variety of detailed information along larger samples of patients. The resulting opt-in status among providers included in quality-improvement registries should be evaluated with caution because it can lead to potential bias for select research questions.[50,51] For the foreseeable future, however, quality-improvement data collection is one of the mandatory pay-for-performance targets in the Centers for Medicare and Medicaid Services (CMS) Merit-based Incentive Payment System, which may drive increased participation in quality-improvement registries and/or development of new specialty-specific quality-improvement registries.[52]

Patient/Disease Registries

Registries that track patients according to their disease or injury, such as the Surveillance, Epidemiology, and End Results (SEER) cancer registry and National Trauma Data Bank (NTDB), traditionally have been organized by diagnosis or exposure (eg, cancer or trauma, respectively) and not treatment received (eg, hand surgery).[9,26,27] Many of these registries contain broad national samples, are relatively inexpensive, and may be easily linked to other sources of secondary data (eg, SEER-Medicare). Sampling design (ie, voluntary participation) and data sources (eg, claims and inpatient facilities), how-ever, are variable and must be considered when choosing the appropriate registry for a specific study question.

The distinguishing benefit of patient/disease registries versus other sources of secondary data is the collection of additional information specific to the cohort of interest (eg, cancer-specific details for SEER data). This feature is important for hand surgery research, because it necessitates collection of specific data that typi-cally are not included in other types secondary data. Also, patient/disease registries that eval-uate data within a specific subspecialty (eg, hand surgery) also may be used for quality improvement and provider performance.[53–55] The UK National Hand Registry, the Swedish Na-tional Healthcare Quality Registry for Hand Sur-gery, and the Surgical Outcomes System in the United States all are good examples of this, and their ability to inform health services research in hand surgery surely will grow in the coming years.[53–55]

CHALLENGES ASSOCIATED WITH PERFORMING SECONDARY DATA RESEARCH IN HAND SURGERY

Hand surgery is a diverse field that is different from other surgical specialties and subsequently faces distinct challenges and limitations when performing secondary data analyses. Relevant history and physical examination findings in hand surgery are unique and not available in most data. Similarly, indications for surgery and timing of surgical intervention for many elective hand procedures depend on functional, social, and patient convenience factors that are not readily measured or documented in medical re-cords. Finally, many outcomes of interest are dependent on availability and access to outside physical and occupational therapy services that typically are not measured or easily linked to existing data sets.

In addition to the absence of relevant data for meaningful health services research, a majority of hand surgery procedures are able to be per-formed in a wide variety of clinical settings, mak-ing it difficult to isolate comprehensive patient cohorts in a single data set. Therefore, hand sur-gery health services researchers must be extremely resourceful in evaluating multiple sour-ces of data sources and well-versed in data link-age to perform impactful secondary data analyses. An algorithm to evaluate potential sec-ondary data research questions in hand surgery is provided.

ALGORITHM TO EVALUATE POTENTIAL SECONDARY DATA RESEARCH QUESTIONS IN HAND SURGERY
Step 1: Define Research Question and Data Needs

The first step for any research study is to clearly define the research question and recognize the potential impact of study conclusions. This is especially important for health services research that requires data safety agreements with payers or health care organizations to obtain necessary data (eg, identifiable claims data). For hand sur-gery, stakeholder collaboration also may be a use-ful way to obtain critical data that otherwise would be unavailable (physical/occupational therapy claims, workers compensation reports, and so forth).

Prior to obtaining data, researchers must iden-tify the required levels of data (eg, patient, hospital, and geographic region) and variables of interest at each data level to study their proposed research question. Drafting a conceptual model of the research question is helpful during this process to identify factors that contribute to the proposed research question and evaluate the potential rela-tionships of these variables to each other.[17] Re-searchers then must identify the unit of observation for their proposed analysis in order to understand the manner in which the existing data sources may need to be manipulated prior to analysis.

Step 2: Identify Potential Sources of Data and Evaluate Data Limitations

Once the research question and data needs have been defined, researchers should evaluate all po-tential sources of data that contain the variables of interest. **Table 2** provides an outline of key con-cepts and statistical considerations when evalu-ating secondary data sources for specific research questions. Often, a single data set is insufficient to address the study needs and linkage is desired for comprehensive analysis. To assess the potential for linkage, researchers should consider the cost of additional data, type of link-age (direct vs indirect) needed, and the coding re-sources required to link the data. If linkage is not feasible, researchers should understand how the absence of linked data will have an impact on the validity of their results and potentially modify their study question or adjust their cohort to fit within these limitations. For example, if a researcher wants to study flexor tendon repairs af-ter trauma but only has access to the NTDB that does not have CPT procedure codes or follow-up information, the researcher may address these

Table 2
Key concepts to consider when evaluating limitations of secondary data sources

Concept	Comments and Statistical Considerations
Data Characteristics: • Identifiable • Level • Type/Source	• Majority of data is de-identified to protect patient privacy • Patient identifiable information is more expensive and difficult to obtain but allows linkage to other data sources • Statistical analysis requires data that is at the same level, therefore data at different levels must be manipulated through patient/hospital level identifiers prior to analysis • Understanding why and how the data was collected may lend insight regarding potential bias in data reporting, accuracy, consistency
Data Sampling Methods • Patient inclusion/exclusion criteria • Data collection process • Participation criteria	• Evaluate whether the dataset has the capacity to study the population of interest in the appropriate clinical setting of care • Often, the patient sample does not match the population of interest and various statistical techniques (e.g., weighting, methods to account for clustering) may be required to accurately generalize study conclusions • Voluntary or restricted sampling methods (e.g., limited insurance carriers, select universities, or participation fees) may contain biased populations that cannot be addressed with statistical methods
Ability to Measure Outcome of Interest • ICD vs. CPT • Cost vs. Charge • Duration of Available Data	• Hospital coding (ICD-9/10) is not as relevant/detailed as provider coding (CPT) for surgical procedures and limits the ability to narrow study populations • Many hospital-based discharge data include hospital charge data that is not as relevant/accurate as payment data (billing claims) and requires application of cost-to-charge ratios to approximate cost • Cost/charge data should be adjusted for inflation in studies >1 year
Ability to Measure Explanatory Variables • Unmeasured Factors • Suitability of Proxy Variables • Relationship Among Explanatory Variables	• It is critical to develop a conceptual model that identifies and characterizes all potential factors that may contribute to the research question • Unmeasured factors may be addressed by linking other data sources or identifying potential proxy variables that are closely associated with the variable of interest • It is important to consider changes in variable construction over time • Statistical analysis should also account for correlation (collinearity) among explanatory variables of interest and clustering (nesting) of multi-level data
Data quality • Missing data (frequency, random/biased) • Coding changes	• Missing data should be examined and characterized (frequency and randomness) for each variable prior to statistical analysis • Whenever possible, missing data should be imputed prior to analysis • It is important to understand coding changes (ICD-9/10, CPT) that occurred over the duration of study and how this may impact the quality of data collection • Many datasets undergo changes in data collection and entry over time, which needs to be accounted for when assessing trends

limitations in several ways: (1) refine the study question to accommodate patient/treatment identification with *International Classification of Disease* (ICD), *Ninth Revision*, and *ICD, Tenth Revision (ICD-9/10)* diagnosis and procedure codes; (2) limit the sample to a single institution or health system and use unique identifiers to link data to the electronic medical record; or (3) develop a probabilistic linkage algorithm to link the data set to another data source using common variables.[56]

Once a data set for a specific research question is selected, researchers should understand the nuances of each variable, how the data were collected, and changes in the data collection method/variable characterization over the course of the study period. Hand surgery health services researchers should pay careful attention to sampling methods, settings of care, and availability of sampling weights to generalize their conclusions. This is because hand surgery cases usually are under-represented in most data sets and the data set setting of care may not match the usual setting of care for a specific hand surgery procedure. An example of this, using the case discussed previously, is that many flexor tendon injuries are not treated in the acute inpatient hospital setting. Therefore, any flexor tendon injuries captured in this data set may not be representative of the overall population. Furthermore, even if the scope of the study is adjusted to include inpatients only, the use of sampling weights is required to compensate for the small and likely unbalanced patient population that is identified.

Step 3: Identify Methods to Reduce Data Limitations

Every secondary data analysis has data limitations. Given the inherent issues of small sample size, variation in clinical setting, and detailed clinical information required to perform secondary data analysis in hand surgery, it is critical for hand surgeons performing this research to be trained rigorously in statistical methods to reduce data limitations. Although a comprehensive review of all statistical techniques used with secondary data is beyond the scope of this article, a few key techniques that the authors believe will become increasingly important as the number and scope of secondary data sources continue to expand are reviewed.

The ability to link (direct and indirect) and aggregate data from different sources is a critical skill for hand surgeons performing research using secondary data. This includes methods of variable preparation (reverse coding, dummy variables, and so forth), imputation of missing data (when possible), and evaluation of variable collinearity. Similarly, researchers should familiarize themselves with multilevel statistical methods and techniques to account for clustering of patients within hospitals or insurance groups and of hospitals within geographic regions or policy boundaries. Finally, as patient-reported outcomes and survey data become readily available on a large scale, applying statistical methods to psychometric data (eg, factor analysis) will become more important.

Step 4: Assess Payment/Policy Implications

Once the analysis has been performed, researchers should consider how their results have an impact on current payment policy. A recent article by Clancy and colleagues[57] states that health services research can influence policy in 4 ways: (1) identifying critical problems, (2) researching the benefits and arms of policy solutions, (3) estimating the costs and consequences of policy proposals, and (4) actively participating in the policy process to aid real-time decision making. For health services research to best influence policy, it is essential to engage stakeholders early in the research process and communicate findings to a diverse group of colleagues and decision makers with different backgrounds. Although several policy-relevant, peer-reviewed journals have accelerated paths for publishing articles that address a timely issue, many surgical journals do not, and proceeding with publication in these journals may result in missing a critical policy window. Furthermore, many policymakers do not have backgrounds in medicine or surgery and do not read research published in traditional surgical journals.

Engaging and collaborating with stakeholders are critical to maximizing potential research impact. Researchers should be aware, however, that successful partnership and data acquisition also may result in alteration of the initial research goal to meet the contextual needs of the policy partner. For example, a hand surgery researcher initially interested in studying access to finger replantation under the Emergency Medical Treatment and Labor Act may need to expand evaluation to all emergency room visits requiring a hand or microvascular surgeon because the stakeholder partner is interested primarily in studying specialist availability. Hand surgery researchers engaging with policy partners should be willing to collaborate with other specialties to assess common general conditions that may be of greater interest to the particular stakeholder.

SUMMARY AND FUTURE RECOMMENDATIONS

Compared with other surgical specialties, hand surgery is a relatively small and unique field. The care provided to patients is critical for their function and quality of life but easily overlooked within the context of currently collected data sets. The distinct preoperative factors, physical examination findings, and postoperative care required to deliver high-value care in hand surgery necessitate specialized data collection and organization that will become increasingly important in the era of value-based payment reform.

As the role of secondary data in surgical research continues to expand and inform quality/performance measure design and payment policy, it is incumbent on all hand surgeons involved in health services research to educate themselves regarding the limitations of current secondary data sources and develop strategies to overcome these issues moving forward. First and foremost, hand surgery needs to substantially invest in data-sharing resources and research programs to leverage existing data sources and identify areas of weakness. Next, surgeons should develop collaborative patient registries to overcome existing data limitations and also satisfy increasing CMS quality-reporting requirements. Finally, hand surgery also needs to foster educational programs to train health services researchers in the field so they able to effectively collaborate with stakeholders and conduct impactful research that best reflects the value of care provided to patients and other providers in the context of the overall health system.

DISCLOSURE

The authors have nothing to disclose.

REFERENCES

1. Ramanathan T, Schmit C, Menon A, et al. The role of law in supporting secondary uses of electronic health information. J Law Med Ethics 2015;43(0 1): 48–51.
2. Centers for Medicare and Medicaid Services Quality Payment Program. Available at: https://qpp.cms.gov/. Accessed September 30, 2019.
3. Quality Programs American College of Surgeons. Available at: https://www.facs.org/quality-programs. Accessed September 30, 2019.
4. Healthcare cost and utilization project databases. Available at: https://www.hcup-us.ahrq.gov/databases.jsp. Accessed September 30, 2019.
5. Research data assistance center. Available at: https://www.resdac.org. Accessed September 30, 2019.
6. Centers for Medicare and Medicaid Services. Research, statistics, data & systems. Available at: https://www.cms.gov/Research-Statistics-Data-and-Systems/Research-Statistics-Data-and-Systems.html. Accessed September 30, 2019.
7. Agency for healthcare research and quality CAHPS patient experience surveys and guidance. Available at: https://www.ahrq.gov/cahps/surveys-guidance/index.html. Accessed September 30, 2019.
8. California Office of Statewide Health Planning and Development (OSHPD). Data and reports. Available at: https://oshpd.ca.gov/data-and-reports/. Accessed September 30, 2019.
9. Gliklich R, Dreyer N, Leavy M, editors. Registries for evaluating patient outcomes: a user's guide, Two volumes, Third edition. Rockville, MD: Agency for Healthcare Research and Quality; 2014 (Prepared by the Outcome DEcIDE Center [Outcome Sciences, Inc., a Quintiles company] under Contract No. 290 2005 00351 TO7.) AHRQ Publication No. 13(14)-EHC111. Available at: http://www.effectivehealthcare.ahrq.gov/ registries-guide-3.cfm.
10. Workman TA. Engaging patients in information sharing and data collection: the role of patient-powered registries and research networks. Rockville (MD): Agency for Healthcare Research and Quality; 2013. AHRQ Community Forum White Paper. AHRQ Publication No. 13-EHC124-EF.
11. Haider AH, Bilimoria KY, Kibbe MR. A checklist to elevate the science of surgical database research. JAMA Surg 2018;153(6):505–7.
12. Cole AP, Friedlander DF, Trinh QD. Secondary data sources for health services research in urologic oncology. Urol Oncol 2018;36(4):165–73.
13. Pugely AJ, Martin CT, Harwood JL, et al. Database and registry research in orthopaedic surgery: part 1: claims-based data. J Bone Joint Surg Am 2015; 97(15):1278–87.
14. Pugely AJ, Martin CT, Harwood JL, et al. Database and registry research in orthopaedic surgery: part 2: clinical registry data. J Bone Joint Surg Am 2015;97(21):1799–808.
15. Mahmoudi E, Malay S, Maroukis BL, et al. The application of medicare data for musculoskeletal research in the United States: a systematic review. J Am Acad Orthop Surg 2019;27(13):e622–32.
16. Riley GF. Administrative and claims records as sources of health care cost data. Med Care 2009;47(7 Suppl 1):S51–5.
17. Kaji AH, Rademaker AW, Hyslop T. Tips for analyzing large data sets from the JAMA surgery statistical editors. JAMA Surg 2018;153(6): 508–9.

18. Schlomer BJ, Copp HL. Secondary data analysis of large data sets in urologic oncology: successes and errors to avoid. J Urol 2014;191(3):587–96.

19. Sun M, Lipsitz SR. Comparative effectiveness research methodology using secondary data: a starting user's guide. Urol Oncol 2018;36(4):174–82.

20. Cole AP, Trinh Q-D. Secondary data analysis: techniques for comparing interventions and their limitations. Curr Opin Urol 2017;27(4):354–9.

21. Dimick JB, Ghaferi AA. Practical guide to surgical data sets: medicare claims data. JAMA Surg 2018; 153(7):677–8.

22. Mahmoudi E, Kotsis S, Chung KC. A review of the use of medicare claims data in plastic surgery outcomes research. Plast Reconstr Surg Glob Open 2015;3(10):e530.

23. Raval MV, Pawlik TM. Practical guide to surgical data sets: National Surgical Quality Improvement Program (NSQIP) and pediatric NSQIP. JAMA Surg 2018;153(8):764–5.

24. Stulberg JJ, Haut ER. Practical guide to surgical data sets: healthcare cost and utilization project National Inpatient Sample (NIS). JAMA Surg 2018; 153(6):586–7.

25. Schoenfeld AJ, Kaji AH, Haider AH. Practical guide to surgical data sets: military health system tricare encounter data. JAMA Surg 2018;153(7):679–80.

26. Hashmi ZG, Kaji AH, Nathens AB. Practical guide to surgical datasets: National Trauma Data Bank (NTDB). JAMA Surg 2018;153(9):852–3.

27. Doll KM, Rademaker A, Sosa JA. Practical guide to surgical data sets: Surveillance, Epidemiology, and End Results (SEER) database. JAMA Surg 2018; 153(6):588–9.

28. Massarweh NN, Kaji AH, Itani KM. Practical guide to surgical data sets: Veterans Affairs Surgical Quality Improvement Program (VASQIP). JAMA Surg 2018; 153(8):768–9.

29. Merkow RP, RAdemaker AW, Billimoria KY. Practical guide to surgical data sets: National Cancer Database (NCDB). JAMA Surg 2018;153(9):850–1.

30. Squitieri L, Russell TA, Ko CY. When one data set is insufficient- things to consider when linking secondary data. JAMA Surg 2019;154(2):186–7.

31. Research Data Assistance Center (ResDAC). Strengths and limitations of CMS administrative data in research. Available at: https://www.resdac.org/articles/strengths-and-limitations-cms-administrative-data-research. Accessed September 30, 2019.

32. Lawson EH, Louie R, Zingmond DS, et al. A comparison of clinical registry versus administrative claims data for reporting of 30-day surgical complications. Ann Surg 2012;256:973–81.

33. Smith S, Snyder A, McMahon LF, et al. Success in hospital-acquired pressure ulcer prevention: a tale in two data sets. Health Aff (Millwood) 2018;37(11): 1787–96.

34. Romano PS, Mark DH. Bias in the coding of hospital discharge data and its implications for quality assessment. Med Care 1994;32:81–90.

35. Squitieri L, Ganz DA, Mangione CM, et al. Consistency of pressure injury documentation across interfacility transfers. BMJ Qual Saf 2018;27(3): 182–9.

36. Song Y, Skinner J, Bynum J, et al. Regional variations in diagnostic practices. N Engl J Med 2010; 363:45–53.

37. Finkelstein A, Gentzkow M, Hull P, et al. Adjusting risk adjustment – accounting for variation in diagnostic intensity. N Engl J Med 2017;376(7):608–10.

38. PearlDiver Healthcare Research. Available at: http://www.pearldiverinc.com. Accessed September 30, 2019.

39. IBM MarketScan Research. Available at: https://marketscan.truvenhealth.com/marketscanportal/. Accessed September 30, 19.

40. Healthcare cost and utilization project quality control procedures. Available at: https://www.hcup-us.ahrq.gov/db/quality.jsp#procedures. Accessed September 30, 2019.

41. MIT Critical Data, editor. Secondary Analysis of Electronic Health Records. 1st edition. Heidelberg (Germany): Springer International Publishing; 2016.

42. PCORNet. The National Patient-Centered Clinical Research Network. Available at: https://pcornet.org. Accessed September 30, 2019.

43. Edgcomb JB, Zima B. Machine learning, natural language processing, and the electronic health record: innovations in mental health services research. Psychiatr Serv 2019;70(4):346–9.

44. Wagaw F, Okoro CA, Kim S, et al. Linking data from health surveys and electronic health records: a demonstration project in two Chicago Health Center Clinics. Prev Chronic Dis 2018;15:E09.

45. West SL, Johnson W, Visscher W, et al. The challenges of linking health insurer claims with electronic medical records. Health Informatics J 2014;20(1): 22–34.

46. Agency for Healthcare Research and Quality. Medical expenditure panel survey. Available at: https://www.meps.ahrq.gov/mepsweb/. Accessed September 30, 2019.

47. National Center for Health Statistics. National health interview survey. Available at: https://www.cdc.gov/nchs/nhis/index.htm. Accessed September 30, 2019.

48. Billimoria KY, Chung JW, Hedges LV, et al. National cluster-randomized trial of duty-hour surgical training. N Engl J Med 2016;374:713–27.

49. Lawson EH, Ko CY, Louie R, et al. Linkage of a clinical surgical registry with medicare inpatient claims data using indirect identifiers. Surgery 2013;153(3): 423–30.

50. Rowell KS, Turrentine FE, Hutter MM, et al. Use of national surgical quality improvement program data as a catalyst for quality improvement. J Am Coll Surg 2007;204(6):1293–300.

51. Osborne NH, Nicholas LH, Ryan AM, et al. Association of hospital participation in a quality reporting program with surgical outcomes and expenditures for medicare beneficiaries. JAMA 2015;313(5): 496–504.

52. Printz C. MACRA paves way for changes in reimbursements: physicians hopeful law will lead to more value-based care. Cancer 2015;121: 2103–4.

53. Arner M. Developing a national quality registry for hand surgery: challenges and opportunities. EFORT Open Rev 2016;1(4):100–6.

54. Surgical outcomes system. Available at: https://surgicaloutcomesystem.com/. Accessed September 30, 2019.

55. British Society of Surgery for the Hand. UK National Hand Registry (Formerly the Audit Database). Available at: https://www.bssh.ac.uk/about/news. Accessed September 30, 2019.

56. Kessinger M, Kumar RB, Ritter AC, et al. A probabilistic matching approach to link de-identified data from a trauma registry and traumatic brain injury model system center. Am J Phys Med Rehabil 2017;96(1):17–24.

57. Clancy CM, Glied SA, Lurie N. From research to health policy impact. Health Serv Res 2012;47(1 Pt 2):337–43.

Providing Hand Surgery Care to Vulnerably Uninsured Patients

Christina I. Brady, MD[a], James M. Saucedo, MD, MBA[b],*

KEYWORDS

- Hand surgery • Indigent care • Unfunded at-risk patient • Safety-net hospital
- Social determinants of health • Poverty • Affordable Medical Care Act • Medicaid

KEY POINTS

- Vulnerable populations are defined in the United States as those at increased risk of poor health because of poor social determinants of health; they can include both the unfunded and underfunded.
- Safety-net hospitals are critical for addressing health care disparities and challenges facing indigent patients.
- Institutions and physicians with articulated altruistic missions are more successful in providing care to indigent patients.

IDENTIFYING VULNERABLE POPULATIONS

The true measure of any society can be found in how it treats its most vulnerable members.
— Mahatma Gandhi[a]

The term vulnerable can be challenging to define, because it often conjures up a myriad of images that clinicians confront in the news, their communities, their practices, and sometimes in their own experiences. In research, vulnerable populations are defined as those who may have difficulty providing voluntary informed consent because of limitations in decision-making capacity or situational circumstances.[1] Vulnerable groups can include racial and ethnic minorities, institutionalized individuals, children, those with chronic illnesses, and those who live in poverty.[2] In health care, many of those same risk factors can also negatively affect clinical outcomes.[2,3]

Although significant progress has been made in protecting vulnerable populations in research, clinicians continue to debate how best to care for many of those same populations when it comes to safety-net and social welfare programs. Some of the more polarizing issues for the last 10 years have pertained to health care and not just how, but even whether, society is responsible for providing health care to anyone who needs it. During this ongoing debate, clinicians continue to struggle with issues of defining eligibility, access, quality, and how to pay for it.

Before the Affordable Care Act (ACA), 44 million nonelderly Americans were estimated to be without medical insurance. After the major coverage provisions went into effect, that number continued to decrease to less than 27 million in 2016. However, in 2017, the number of uninsured people increased by nearly 700,000 people, the first increase since the implementation of the ACA.[4] Although the number of people without health insurance has decreased, access to health care resources

[a] Department of Orthopaedic Surgery, UT Health San Antonio, MC-7774, 7703 Floyd Curl Drive, San Antonio, TX 78229, USA; [b] Orthopedics & Sports Medicine, Houston Methodist Hospital, 13802 Centerfield Drive, Suite 300, Houston, TX 77070, USA
* Corresponding author.
E-mail addresses: James.Saucedo.MD@gmail.com; jsaucedo@houstonmethodist.org

[a]Forms of this quote have been attributed to other figures in history as well.

Hand Clin 36 (2020) 245–253
https://doi.org/10.1016/j.hcl.2020.01.013

remains a problem. However, health insurance does not in itself guarantee access to appropriate care in a reasonable time frame.

Perhaps as important as defining those without health insurance is to identify those who are under-insured. In 2005, a Commonwealth Fund study defined underinsured as those whose "out-of-pocket health care costs, excluding premiums, were at least 10 percent of their income, or 5 percent if their income was less than 200 percent of poverty ($22,980 for an individual in a 2014 plan)… [as well as those] whose health insurance deductibles were at least 5 percent of their income."[5] Of the 194 million US adults aged 19 to 64 years in 2018, an estimated 87 million, or 45%, were found to be inadequately insured.[6] These are patients who, despite having health insurance on paper, are not always able to access the care they need in a timely manner.

However, it is not just Americans who are without insurance or even only those who have bare-bone plans with high premiums who are at risk. A federal report on the economic well-being of US households in 2017 found that 4 in 10 adults, if faced with an unexpected expense of $400, would either not be able to cover it or would cover it by selling something or borrowing money. In addition, more than one-fourth of adults skipped necessary medical care in 2017 because of being unable to afford the cost.[7] Depending on how vulnerable is defined, the group of people to whom this applies may be bigger than is often thought. If a more inclusive definition of vulnerable is used, it may even show that it includes a significant portion of US communities and readers may find that it includes someone they know.

Evaluating vulnerable patients in society also involves identifying their relative risk of poor health.[3] Aside from health insurance or the ability to pay for it, some patients are at a higher risk simply because of being poor. Poor social determinants of health include poverty, low education or limited health literacy, physical environment, and limited access to health care[8] (**Fig. 1**). Accordingly, successful initiatives to provide hand surgery care to vulnerable uninsured patients will need to address not only the financial component but also other underlying relative social determinants of health that can affect patients' health outcomes.

There are several national programs worth acknowledging that successfully capture and deliver care to certain identified vulnerable populations, including Medicaid, Indian Health Services, Veterans Administration, and Medicare. Nonetheless, there are additional vulnerable populations who have not been completely covered by national safety-net programs. These populations include healthy young men without employer-based health insurance and undocumented immigrants. Such patients are often employed in manual labor jobs and have a particular dependence on their hands for employment, which places hand surgeons on the front line of caring for such injuries.

Although work-related injuries may be generally covered by workers' compensation plans, non–work-related injuries can be potentially devastating, especially for undocumented immigrants. These patients do not qualify for federal coverage, such as Medicaid, and are not allowed to participate in the insurance exchange.[9] A lack of resources makes safety-net hospitals and free clinics especially important to these populations

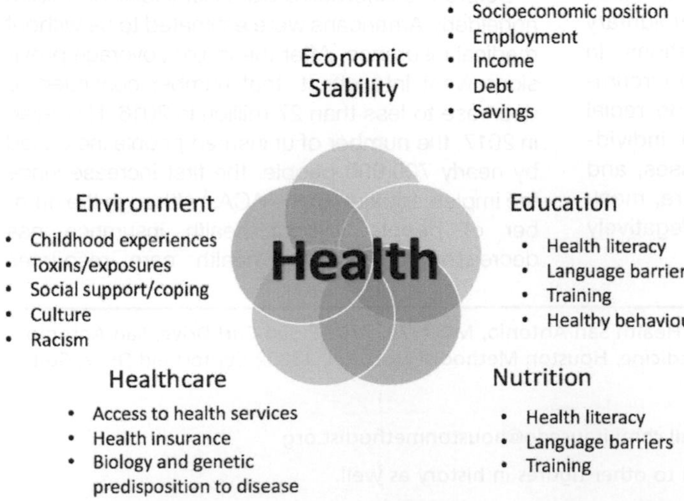

Economic Stability
- Socioeconomic position
- Employment
- Income
- Debt
- Savings

Environment
- Childhood experiences
- Toxins/exposures
- Social support/coping
- Culture
- Racism

Education
- Health literacy
- Language barriers
- Training
- Healthy behaviours

Healthcare
- Access to health services
- Health insurance
- Biology and genetic predisposition to disease

Nutrition
- Health literacy
- Language barriers
- Training

Health

Fig. 1. Contributing factors to the social determinants of health.

and others who may not be aware of or eligible for other programs.

DIRECT AND INDIRECT COSTS OF INDIGENT CARE

There are significant financial risks attributable to the direct and indirect costs of providing care for vulnerable patients, including costs to the patient themselves, their providers, and society as a whole through government agencies and other institutions. Even with the implementation of the ACA, medical costs remain the number 1 reason why Americans file for bankruptcy.[10] For uninsured patients, unforeseen trauma leads to catastrophic health expenditures in 7 out of 10 patients.[11] For example, if a 26-year-old male manual laborer with an annual wage of $36,590 sustains a brachial plexus injury, his short-term wage loss is estimated to be $22,740, whereas the long-term wage loss may be close to $737,551.00. In his postinjury lifetime, the mean indirect cost from such an injury is calculated to be $1,113,962.[12]

In addition to the patients, hospitals and providers often bear the cost of the care they provide to unfunded patients. For example, one study that focused on a level 2 trauma center found that the mean charge for patients was $162,152.00, with a mean length of stay of 13.2 days. For the 128 patients included in the study over 4 years, the total charges amounted to $4.5 million, with reimbursement of just less than $1 million.[13] Such a shortfall between expenses and reimbursement can place an unsustainable burden on the providers, communities, and small hospital systems that care for unfunded patients. Overall in the United States, uncompensated costs of care for the uninsured totaled $84.9 billion in 2013. Of that sum, $53.3 billion was paid to hospitals and providers to help offset costs, most of which came from the federal government. Uninsured patients paid an additional $25.8 billion in out-of-pocket costs for their care.[14]

ETHICAL OBLIGATION TO CHARITY CARE

One of the dilemmas for surgeons and providers, particularly in private practice, is the moral and ethical obligation to care for indigent patients even when reimbursement is not guaranteed. Although the hospital may recoup costs associated with caring for these patients through charitable and governmental funding, contracted surgeons may never be reimbursed for procedures they perform while taking call. This possibility

sometimes leads to the practice of "cherry-picking" patients, which may result in a higher distribution of burden to safety-net hospitals and other providers in the community.[15,16] In such situations, there remains the question of who carries the ethical obligation of charity care.

The burden to provide care for indigent patients has been included in the American Medical Association Code of Medical Ethics since 1847. However, when it was rewritten in 1947, there was a shift of burden toward larger institutions:

The poverty of a patient and the mutual obligation of physicians should command the gratuitous services of a physician. But endowed institutions and organizations for mutual benefit, or for accident, sickness and life insurance, or for analogous purposes, have no claim upon physicians for unremunerated services.[17]

In other words, although physicians are expected to care for patients regardless of their ability to pay, endowed institutions (those who receive funding for this purpose) should help support physicians in that mission and should not expect physicians to incur financial harm as a result.

BARRIERS TO HEALTH CARE FOR VULNERABLE PATIENTS

In 1971, Julian Tudor Hart[18] coined the phrase inverse care law to describe a paradox he observed in which the availability of medical or social care varied inversely with the need of the population. He notes that susceptibility to this phenomenon increases in areas where medical care is most exposed to market forces.[18] This phenomenon is especially clear in the United States, where income has been found to be directly correlated to life expectancy, with a difference of 14.6 years for men and 10.1 years for women between the wealthiest 1% and the poorest 1%.[19]

The barriers that indigent patients encounter frequently extend beyond a lack of access to health care. In addition to the financial obstacles of direct and indirect costs, patients may also face cultural barriers, such as negative cultural attitudes toward medicine or fears of surgery. There are also structural barriers, such as access to subspecialists.[20] In addition, limited health literacy is an often underappreciated but substantial barrier to effective communication with patients. Patients with limited health literacy have been observed to ask fewer questions regarding their medical care during visits with hand surgeons,[21] which may have a detrimental effect on their acceptance of or adherence to certain treatment recommendations.

In addition, mental and psychological comorbidities may go unrecognized and complicate the clinical picture. In indigent patients undergoing a total knee arthroplasty, screening for underlying mental disorder revealed that 35% of those patients had an axis-1 psychological disorder. In these patients, perceived outcome scores at 1 year were lower even despite an improvement in overall function.[22]

In caring for indigent patients at her institution, one of the authors observed recurrent challenges, including but not limited to delay in presentation, lack of social support, inability to take time off from work to recover, transportation issues, language barriers, higher risk of loss to follow-up, and higher substance abuse issues. Often, these social issues prove to be more significant obstacles to recovery than their surgical condition. However, insurance-related differences only add to the baseline risk for worse surgical outcomes.[23]

MEDICAID AND SAFETY-NET HOSPITALS

In 1965, President Lyndon B. Johnson signed Medicaid and Medicare into law as amendments to the Social Security Act. Medicaid programs have evolved to become a major component of the United States' solution to meeting the challenges of the vulnerable uninsured. As an income-based health coverage program for low-income individuals, Medicaid has expanded since 1965 to increase the number of beneficiaries. In 1997, the Children's Health Insurance Program was enacted to ensure coverage for children up to at least 200% of the federal poverty level (FPL). Then, in 2010, as part of the ACA, Medicaid benefits were expanded to nonelderly adults with income up to 138% of the FPL ($17,236 for individuals in 2019).

Although there are stipulations tied to federal funding for Medicaid programs, the state governments decide how to deliver Medicaid care to their constituents. The adoption of the ACA was determined to be state-dependent by a 2012 Supreme Court ruling, and states were given a choice to accept or defer the expansion of Medicaid funding. For this reason, Medicaid programs can vary between states. In 2017, Medicaid covered more than 75 million low-income Americans. Of Medicaid enrollees, 43% are children, and elderly patients and those with disabilities account for around 25% of enrollees.[24]

As mentioned earlier, insurance coverage in itself does not guarantee access to care, making safety-net hospitals the mainstay of providing health care for individuals regardless of their ability to pay. From a practical standpoint, they are an invaluable asset for the community through the care they provide as well as their economic contributions. In 2017, safety-net hospitals provided $6.7 billion in uncompensated care, which represents 17.4% of the uncompensated care nationally. Economically, safety-net hospitals employ, on average, 3072 people and provide $1.1 billion to the state economy per hospital.[20] They also provide the foundation for training future physicians. In discussing ways to provide care for uninsured vulnerable populations, preservation of resources for safety-net hospitals needs to remain a top priority.

Overall, the expansion of Medicaid through the ACA has had a positive financial impact on safety-net hospitals. In states that expanded Medicaid, there was an increase in Medicaid inpatient days and Medicaid revenues along with a decrease in uncompensated care costs. However, states that did not accept the Medicaid expansion did not see this positive effect.[25] There was also a decrease in the likelihood of closure of hospitals, specifically in rural markets, in states that expanded Medicaid.[26]

In patients with trauma hospitalized across 11 Medicaid expansion states, there was an 18.2% increase in Medicaid coverage and a 15.1% decrease in uninsured patients. There was no significant difference in patient mortality or unplanned readmission rates, and discharge to rehabilitation centers increased by 1.2%.[27] Specifically, in hand surgery, the ACA has led to a decrease in the proportion of uninsured patients with an increase in Medicaid coverage. However, despite the increase in coverage, overall physician reimbursement did not change. The lackluster improvement in overall reimbursement may be attributed to unexpected decreases in reimbursement rates,[28] which may have in effect counterbalanced the increased volume of covered patients. Though perhaps disappointing, it is important to acknowledge that more people had access to care without an absolute decrease in compensation for providers.

Participation in the Medicaid expansion does not seem to be the only way to secure funding for safety-net hospitals. Texas and Florida did not expand Medicaid eligibility under the ACA but were able to secure additional funding through Medicaid waivers. States can obtain Section 1115 demonstration waivers, which allow states to waive certain federal restrictions for Medicaid funding. Shortly after the change in administrations, the Centers for Medicare and Medicaid Services (CMS) approved waivers from Florida and Texas to increase the funding for uncompensated care in the states by 50% to 70%.[29] Expansion of care through Medicaid waivers may provide an alternative strategy for funding the care of uninsured populations.

HOW SAFETY-NET HOSPITALS CAN PREPARE FOR REFORM AND IMPROVE PATIENT CARE

Safety-net hospitals can position themselves to better meet the demands of future funding uncertainty. Evaluation of the 5 leading safety-net hospitals found common themes central to preparing for health care reform[30]:

1. Strong and stable leadership
2. A long-term commitment to improving care and care delivery through investing in information technology
3. Developing integrated systems of care
4. Aligning safety-net and academic missions

These themes overlap with 6 best practices that were identified by a special committee of the Department of Health and Human Services, which was tasked to evaluate distinguishing drivers of quality found in health care systems that were particularly successful in delivering care to at-risk populations. **Fig. 2** shows their best-practice recommendations based on their research.[2]

The transition from a fee-for-service to a value-based payment model will require an honest evaluation of the current practices in health care. Financially driven initiatives without tangible

improvement in patient health outcomes will be challenged by programs that focus on patient-reported outcomes and quality rather than cost or network size. In a quickly changing health care environment, safety-net hospitals should continue adopting strategies to secure ways to prepare for uncertainty with future funding.

SUCCESSFUL EXAMPLES OF CHARITY CARE OUTSIDE OF GOVERNMENT CARE

Altruistic organizations with an articulated commitment to providing care to disadvantaged populations have found ways to continue their missions outside of government programs. Such examples include the Willis-Knighton Health System and the Shriners Hospitals for Children.

Willis-Knighton Health System, a nongovernmental, not-for-profit institution, has successfully delivered care to the underprivileged in Louisiana by looking within its organization for answers. Their formula for sustaining charitable care initiatives revolves around 3 key areas: efficient operation, service line diversification, and a steadfast commitment to serving the disadvantaged.[31]

Shriners, an organization with 22 hospitals for children throughout the United States, Canada, and Mexico, provides state-of-the-art medical care for children with orthopedic disorders and burn injuries. They provide millions of dollars for research and partner with teaching institutions

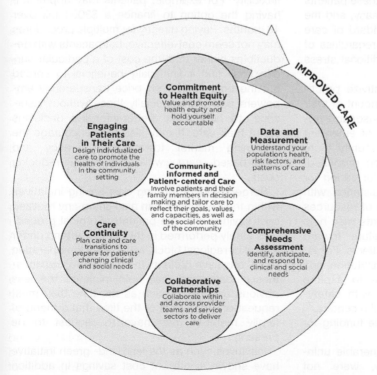

Fig. 2. System practices to improve care for socially at-risk populations. (*From* National Academies of Sciences, Engineering, and Medicine. 2016. Systems practices for the care of socially at-risk populations. Washington, D.C.: The National Academies Press; with permission.)

and other top universities. Through charitable funding, they have provided care for more than 770,000 children over the past 80 years.[32]

These examples show unique but not mutually exclusive approaches to serving their communities. In the case of Willis-Knighton, they have found creative ways to work more efficiently and effectively with what they have, to do more with less, whereas Shriners has developed a fundraising machine to help support their charity's mission. Mission-driven organizations can and will find ways to support that mission in a variety of ways.

SOLUTIONS WITHIN HAND SURGERY PRACTICES TO BETTER ACCOMMODATE INDIGENT PATIENTS

In Atul Gawande's[33] article, "The Cost Conundrum," he concludes that, "The most expensive piece of medical equipment, as the saying goes, is a doctor's pen. And, as a rule, hospital executives don't own the pen caps. Doctors do." Physicians can contribute significantly to improving the system for vulnerable patients. The easiest approach is to first address cost and quality within medical practices. Affordability of care can lead to increased access to medical care for the poor. The commitment from physicians to provide medical services for indigent patients is not only admirable; it remains the most important component of ensuring that the medical needs for these patients are met. However, it is not always easy, and the inability to provide the highest standard of care for all patients when they need it, regardless of their ability to pay, can lead to additional stress and burnout for physicians.[34]

Policies or programs that incentivize practitioners to dedicate even a small amount of their practice to charity care may be a reasonable option to help distribute the burden of emergent indigent care throughout the community more evenly. Innovative ideas have been proposed, including allowing tax deductions for caring for indigent patients or providing assistance with malpractice insurance.[35] Allocation of resources to help the doctors help the patients may help galvanize a positive shift in culture toward providing more care for indigent patients. For individual practices not linked to an institution, one option that might help would be to explore limited or expanded partnerships with safety-net hospitals and/or community health centers.[29] As partnerships are made, available funding for indigent patients may follow.

The health disparities facing vulnerable uninsured populations, unfortunately, were not completely resolved with the expansion of Medicaid. Uninsured patients who suddenly qualify for health coverage through Medicaid may still find themselves unable to access the medical care they need. Medicaid provider participation varies significantly among states, ranging from 40% to 99% of physicians accepting Medicaid.[36] In hand clinic appointments, Medicaid patients are less likely to have outpatient access to care. For example, patients with acute flexor tendon injuries may have a harder time making an appointment, potentially because of a limited number of physicians accepting Medicaid.[37] Although practice structures and challenges may vary, a shared and coordinated commitment within and among practices in a community would go far toward improving the care of indigent patients while sharing the costs that it might entail.

Providing low-cost out-of-pocket options for patients with payment plans may offer another viable alternative for unfunded patients, as well as those with high deductible plans (depending on the plan's provisions). Patients who are directly paying for their care may also benefit from a bundled health care model. The emerging online health care marketplace is an evolving industry that allows patients the transparency to compare prices and pay out of pocket for bundled procedures.[38] Because procedures can represent high costs for patients, financing plans offer welcome flexibility. For example, patients may appreciate having the option to finance a $3000 bill over 48 months. Paying directly for multiple procedures may not seem cost-effective, but patients with deductibles higher than the cost of a particular surgery may find it financially beneficial to spread out the cost. Moreover, price transparency empowers patients, especially those without insurance, to help make better-informed decisions about their care. It may also help encourage the remaining market toward transparency and value-based care, while potentially reducing costs.

Surgeons incorporating cost-saving initiatives within their practices can also share any realized cost savings with the patients. Surgical procedures safely performed in the clinical setting under a local or regional block, rather than the operating room, can save patients the facility fee and anesthesia costs, and may help minimize the less obvious expenses, such as the time they must request off from work or the time that a friend of family member may have to request to be present.

Initiatives such as the lean-and-green initiative have shown significant cost savings in addition to decreasing waste without sacrificing the quality of care.[39,40] These initiatives include performing surgery using wide-awake local anesthesia, no tourniquet (WALANT), which allows surgeries to be performed in a less expensive outpatient setting. In contrast with the operating room, surgical setup can be minimal with a single drape and gloves, and at least 1 study showed equal safety with no appreciable increase in the rate of infection.[40,41] In short, WALANT provides an option that is safe, less expensive, and potentially creates more access to patients with fewer financial resources for the appropriate surgical procedures.

In addition, for providers unable to offer care for indigent patients because of either cost or coverage being restrictive, having a protocol that incorporates available local resources that the staff can share with indigent patients can help assuage some of the frustrations frequently encountered. Such resources may include a referral network or arrangements made with a nearby hand surgeon working within safety-net hospitals or community health centers where the patients can more easily establish care. Also, domestic missions or local charity resources, such as Hand Day through the American Society for Surgery of the Hand, provide 1-day missions for pro

---

Box 1
Ideas for surgeons to improve the delivery of care for at-risk populations

Seek partnerships with safety-net hospitals or community health centers

Incorporate an affordable amount of Medicaid into the practice when possible

Identify and implement cost-efficient processes into the practice; minimizing costs indirectly frees up resources for caring for unfunded and underfunded patients.

Offer cost-transparency options with a reasonable payment plan

Consider introducing common procedures that incorporate lean and green concepts, such as WALANT, into the practice

Commit to and articulate a clear mission for caring for all members of the community

Have a set protocol for referral of patients in need of charity care

Be aware of and participate in local charity missions, including Hand Day through the American Society for Surgery of the Hand (ASSH)

Participate in fundraising initiatives for charity organizations or community clinics

---

bono hand surgery for patients in the community without access to hand care.[42]

SUMMARY

Vulnerable patients are defined by an increased risk of poor health secondary to poor social determinants of health and include uninsured as well as underinsured patient populations. When addressing the disparities and barriers these patients encounter, it is important to consider the associated burdens of cost, access to care, and quality of care. Although the ACA has expanded the number of insured patients through Medicaid, a significant number of patients remain outside its reach, and undocumented immigrants remain a particularly vulnerable population.

Safety-net hospitals have and will be the main source of care for the indigent population, and efforts to improve their sustainability will be paramount, especially as funding becomes more restricted. In addition to governmental funding, private organizations and charity organizations continue to care for a large portion of at-risk patients. They can also provide a successful model for other institutions to follow. Surgeons can incorporate best practices to help care for indigent patients, and an effective place to start is by focusing on reducing costs and, in effect, passing some of those cost savings to the patients, such as through in-office procedures. Other strategies include improving patient communication (especially those with limited health literacy) to help identify and overcome certain barriers to care, as well as an awareness of the available resources through charity, safety-net institutions, and local networks of providers who share a desire to share the care of this population.

In addition, mission-driven organizations tend to be most successful in serving their constituents. Articulating a clear mission and committing to finding ways to accomplishing it often lead to better results, even when the challenges seem insurmountable, and the funding seems to dry up. Caring for the indigent requires first that clinicians commit to it. Once they have done that, they can each find ways to play their part, which may take a variety of forms depending on each situation (**Box 1**).

DISCLOSURE

The authors have no relevant disclosures.

REFERENCES

1. Bracken-Roche D, Bell E, Macdonald ME, et al. The concept of 'vulnerability' in research ethics: an

in-depth analysis of policies and guidelines. Health Res Policy Syst 2017;15(1):8.

2. National Academies of Sciences, Engineering, and Medicine. Systems practices for the care of socially at-risk populations. Washington, DC: The National Academics Press; 2016.

3. Aday LA. Health status of vulnerable populations. Annu Rev Public Health 1994;15:487–509.

4. Kaiser Family Foundation analysis of 2008-2017 American Community Survey (ACS) -ye. Key facts about the uninsured population. Available at: http://files.kff.org/attachment//fact-sheet-key-facts-about-the-uninsured-population. Accessed.

5. Schoen C. Insured but not protected: how many adults are underinsured? Health Affairs Wed Exclusive 2005.

6. Collins SR, Bhupal HK, Doty MM. Health insurance coverage eight years after the ACA: fewer uninsured americans and shorter coverage gaps, but more underinsured. Commonwealth Fund; 2019.

7. System BoGotFR. Report on the economics well-being of U.S. households in 2017. Washington, DC: 2017.

8. Foundation KF. Beyond health care: the role of social determinants in promoting health and health equity. Kaiser Family Foundation; 2018. Available at: https://www.kff.org/disparities-policy/issue-brief/beyond-health-care-the-role-of-social-determinants-in-promoting-health-and-health-equity/. Accessed September 1, 2019.

9. Medicaid.gov. Available at: https://www.medicaid.gov/medicaid/eligibility/index.html. Accessed September 1, 2019.

10. Himmelstein DU, Thorne D, Warren E, et al. Medical bankruptcy in the United States, 2007: results of a national study. Am J Med 2009;122(8):741–6.

11. Scott JW, Raykar NP, Rose JA, et al. Cured into destitution: catastrophic health expenditure risk among uninsured trauma patients in the United States. Ann Surg 2018;267(6):1093–9.

12. Hong TS, Tian A, Sachar R, et al. Indirect cost of traumatic brachial plexus injuries in the United States. J Bone Joint Surg Am 2019;101(16):e80.

13. Kane E, Richman PB, Xu KT, et al. Costs and characteristics of undocumented immigrants brought to a trauma center by border patrol agents in Southern Texas. J Emerg Trauma Shock 2019;12(1):54–7.

14. Coughlin TA, Holahan J, Caswell K, et al. An estimated $84.9 billion in uncompensated care was provided in 2013; ACA payment cuts could challenge providers. Health Aff (Millwood) 2014;33(5):807–14.

15. Thakur NA, Plante MJ, Kayiaros S, et al. Inappropriate transfer of patients with orthopaedic injuries to a Level I trauma center: a prospective study. J Orthop Trauma 2010;24(6):336–9.

16. Friebe I, Isaacs J, Mallu S, et al. Evaluation of appropriateness of patient transfers for hand and microsurgery to a level I trauma center. Hand (N Y) 2013;8(4):417–21.

17. Association AM. The duties of physician to each other and to the profession at large, Compensation Code of Medical Ethics. Chicago: AMA Press; 1947.

18. Hart JT. The inverse care law. Lancet 1971;1(7696):405–12.

19. Chetty R, Stepner M, Abraham S, et al. The Association between income and life expectancy in the United States, 2001-2014. JAMA 2016;315(16):1750–66.

20. Yuan F, Chung KC. Impact of safety net hospitals in the care of the hand-injured patient: a national perspective. Plast Reconstr Surg 2016;138(2):429–34.

21. Menendez ME, van Hoorn BT, Mackert M, et al. Patients with limited health literacy ask fewer questions during office visits with hand surgeons. Clin Orthop Relat Res 2017;475(5):1291–7.

22. Ellis HB, Howard KJ, Khaleel MA, et al. Effect of psychopathology on patient-perceived outcomes of total knee arthroplasty within an indigent population. J Bone Joint Surg Am 2012;94(12):e84.

23. Braveman P, Schaaf VM, Egerter S, et al. Insurance-related differences in the risk of ruptured appendix. N Engl J Med 1994;331(7):444–9.

24. Rudowitz R, Garfield R, Hinton E. 10 things to know about Medicaid: setting the facts straight. Kaiser Family Foundation; 2019. Available at: http://files.kff.org/attachment/Issue-Brief-10-Things-to-Know-about-Medicaid-Setting-the-Facts-Straight. Accessed September 1, 2019.

25. Dobson A, DaVanzo JE, Haught R, et al. Comparing the affordable care act's financial impact on safety-net hospitals in states that expanded Medicaid and those that did not. Issue Brief (Commonw Fund) 2017;2017:1–10.

26. Lindrooth RC, Perraillon MC, Hardy RY, et al. Understanding the relationship between medicaid expansions and hospital closures. Health Aff (Millwood) 2018;37(1):111–20.

27. Akande M, Minneci PC, Deans KJ, et al. Association of Medicaid expansion under the affordable care act with outcomes and access to rehabilitation in young adult trauma patients. JAMA Surg 2018;153(8):e181630.

28. Khansa I, Khansa L, Pearson GD, et al. Effects of the affordable care act on payer mix and physician reimbursement in hand surgery. J Hand Surg Am 2018;43(6):511–5.

29. Kelley AT, Tipirneni R. Care for undocumented immigrants - rethinking state flexibility in medicaid waivers. N Engl J Med 2018;378(18):1661–3.

30. Coughlin TA, Long SK, Sheen E, et al. How five leading safety-net hospitals are preparing for the challenges and opportunities of health care reform. Health Aff (Millwood) 2012;31(8):1690–7.

31. Elrod JK, Fortenberry JL Jr. Bridging access gaps experienced by the underserved: the need for healthcare providers to look within for answers. BMC Health Serv Res 2017;17(Suppl 4):791.

32. Schumacher W. Lessons from the Shriners. Those guys in the funny hats make possible free hospital care for children. Mod Healthc 2005;35(20):24.

33. Gawande A. The cost conundrum. Ann Med 2009.

34. Walden J. An overlooked cause of physician burnout. Fam Pract Manag 2016;23(1):6–7.

35. Gore DR. Paying for the uninsured. WMJ 2013; 112(3):104.

36. Decker SL. In 2011 nearly one-third of physicians said they would not accept new Medicaid patients, but rising fees may help. Health Aff (Millwood) 2012;31(8):1673–9.

37. Draeger RW, Patterson BM, Olsson EC, et al. The influence of patient insurance status on access to outpatient orthopedic care for flexor tendon lacerations. J Hand Surg Am 2014;39(3):527–33.

38. Rosato D. How paying your doctor in cash could save you money. Consumer reports. 2018. Available at: https://www.consumerreports.org/healthcare-costs/how-paying-your-doctor-in-cash-could-save-you-money/.

39. Tighe J, Brown D, Sela Y, et al. Lean and Green: minimizing waste in hand surgery. American Association for Hand Surgery Annual Meeting. Scottsdale, AZ, January 13, 2016.

40. Van Demark RE Jr, Smith VJS, Fiegen A. Lean and green hand surgery. J Hand Surg Am 2018;43(2): 179–81.

41. Leblanc MR, Lalonde DH, Thoma A, et al. Is main operating room sterility really necessary in carpal tunnel surgery? A multicenter prospective study of minor procedure room field sterility surgery. Hand (N Y) 2011;6(1):60–3.

42. Available at: https://www.assh.org/touching-hands/Act-Now/Host-a-Domestic-Mission. Accessed September 1, 2019.

Impact of Health Care Reform on Technology and Innovation

Preethi Kesavan, BS[a], Christopher J. Dy, MD, MPH[b],*

KEYWORDS

- Medical device industry • Medical device innovation • Device regulation
- Comparative effectiveness research • Postmarket surveillance • Premarket approval
- Frugal innovation

KEY POINTS

- Recent health care reforms prioritizing cost reduction and improved patient outcomes have altered medical device innovation and market regulations.
- Value-based payment reforms have cultivated new trends in innovation such as frugal innovation and deinstitutionalization; however, uncertain reimbursement policies have led to a reduction in venture capitalist investment in new technologies.
- Concerns over medical device safety arising from a lenient market approval process has led to increased US Food and Drug Administration regulations, yet this must be balanced with the resulting increased time to market because this may stifle innovation.
- Comparative effectiveness research has recently gained momentum, although application of its findings proves difficult because of the short life cycle of medical devices.

INTRODUCTION

Many aspects of recent health care reform in the United States have affected technology, innovation, and delivery of care. The medical device industry is a substantial component of the health care system. As of 2019, the industry consists of 859 businesses in the United States with revenues totaling to US$41.3 billion.[1] Although these statistics suggest a thriving, diverse playing field, the bulk of the market is actually composed of a few large companies (**Tables 1** and **2**). These companies occupy 1% of the industry yet account for 82% of total assets.[2,3]

By contrast, small companies, with 73% having fewer than 20 employees and less than $1 million in assets, are often acquired by large companies as a result of challenges with securing funding, manufacturing, distribution, and a lack of established relationships with providers. Yet these companies are crucial to the development of new medical technologies and often focus on narrow therapeutic areas.[2,4] Health care policies that create further market barriers for small companies pose the risk of stunting medical innovation.

Before use in patient-care settings, medical devices undergo a multistep product development process (**Fig. 1**). This process begins with product conception and prototyping. In small and startup companies, this stage requires adequate funding, which is typically assumed by venture capitalist (VC) firms and government grants.[2] The product then undergoes verification and validation analyses to ensure that it meets design and market criteria. Once the product has been deemed ready

a Office of Medical Student Research, Washington University School of Medicine, 660 South Euclid Avenue, Campus Box 8077, St. Louis, MO 63110, USA; b Department of Orthopaedic Surgery, Washington University School of Medicine, 660 South Euclid Avenue, Campus Box 8233, St Louis, MO 63110, USA
* Corresponding author.
E-mail address: dyc@wustl.edu
Twitter: @ChrisDyMD (C.J.D.)

Hand Clin 36 (2020) 255–262
https://doi.org/10.1016/j.hcl.2020.01.008
0749-0712/20/© 2020 Elsevier Inc. All rights reserved.

Table 1
Top 10 United States medical device companies by revenue (2017)

	Company	Revenue in Billion US Dollars
1	Medtronic	29.7
2	Johnson & Johnson	26.6
3	General Electric Healthcare	19.1
4	Abbott Laboratories	16.2
5	Cardinal Health	13.5
6	Stryker	12.4
7	Becton Dickinson	12.1
8	Baxter International	10.6
9	Boston Scientific	9
10	Danaher	8.6

Data from Statista. Medical Product Outsourcing. Top 10 U.S. Medical Technology Companies Based on Revenue in 2017 (in Billion U.S. Dollars). July 2018.

for market entrance, it must undergo a premarket approval process regulated by the Food and Drug Administration (FDA), after which it can enter the market and undergo long-term postmarket surveillance.[5]

Health care reforms centered around improved patient outcomes and cost reduction have had a significant impact on the medical device market and device innovation. Changes in VC investment, allocation of R&D funds, and the FDA approval process are among many changes in the industry. The following sections explore the driving forces of these changes and the resulting challenges faced by various stakeholders.

VENTURE CAPITALIST INVESTMENT TRENDS

In the last decade, payment reforms and uncertainties in reimbursements have led to decreased

Table 2
Top 5 global orthopedic device companies by market share (2017)

	Company	Market Share (%)
1	Johnson & Johnson (USA)	24.2
2	Zimmer Biomet (USA)	20.3
3	Stryker (USA)	16.3
4	Medtronic (USA)	8.3
5	Arthrex (Germany)	5.8

Data from Statista. Global Top 10 Companies Based on Orthopedic Medical Technology Market Share in 2017 and 2024. September 2018.

VC investment in medical device companies. Between 2009 and 2014, total VC invested in all industry sectors increased dramatically from $20.3 billion to $39.6 billion. Investment in life science companies, however, decreased from 35.7% to 19.9% of total investment. Overall, medical technology share of total VC investment decreased from 9% in 2009% to 4% in 2014.[6] A larger decline in investment in early-stage life science companies compared with later-stage life science companies was also observed during this time.[7]

In a survey of more than 150 VCs, 40% of respondents stated uncertainties over coverage and reimbursement policies of new products by CMS (cash management services) and private payers as one of the main reasons for hesitation to invest in life science companies.[7] The new model of value-based purchasing favors more clinical evidence, incurring higher costs that discourage VC investment. In addition, VCs find FDA medical device product review to be slow and inconsistent. The total time required to gain FDA approval and insurance coding, coverage, and payment creates delays in return on investment that are unattractive to VCs.

Industry stakeholders have found investment trends to be concerning for future innovation and have called for multiple policy changes to encourage VC investment. One such policy is increased transparency and timely pathways to coding, coverage, and payment for FDA-approved products. Increased government agency funding for startup company R&D has also been suggested.[7]

IMPLICATIONS OF PAYMENT REFORM

The introduction of new payment models that prioritize positive patient outcomes and cost reduction has incentivized providers to seek out low-cost medical devices. This has in turn altered the market for various purchasing powers. For example, in bundled payments, a fixed rate is set in advance for a surgical procedure. This fixed rate includes implantable devices, supplies, and drugs, among others.[8] To improve profit margins, hospitals must negotiate for lower device prices. With hospitals being the largest market for medical device manufacturers (**Fig. 2**), this theoretically would exert a downward pressure on prices that is passed down to suppliers.[9]

Challenges in Cost Reduction

Although reforms in payment models have pushed hospitals to lower costs, medical device cost depends on multiple factors. The ideal forces necessary to control cost in any market are[2,8]:

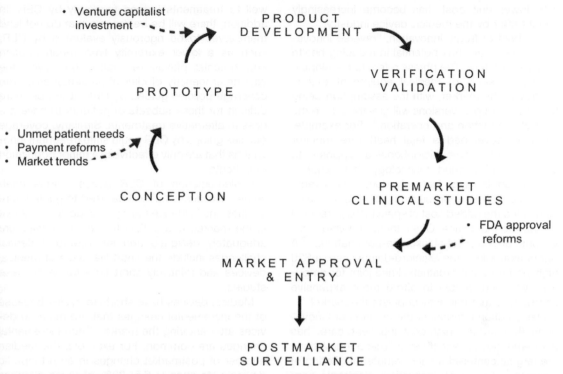

- Venture capitalist investment

PRODUCT DEVELOPMENT

VERIFICATION VALIDATION

PROTOTYPE

- Unmet patient needs
- Payment reforms
- Market trends

PREMARKET CLINICAL STUDIES

CONCEPTION

- FDA approval reforms

MARKET APPROVAL & ENTRY

POSTMARKET SURVEILLANCE

Fig. 1. Medical device development process and factors influencing device innovation.

1. Large number of sellers
2. Existence of similar products in the market
3. Low barriers to entry into the market
4. Transparency in prices, quality, and performance of products

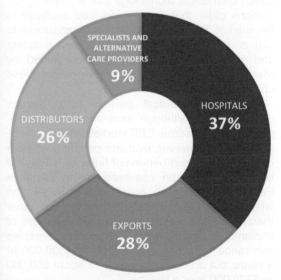

SPECIALISTS AND ALTERNATIVE CARE PROVIDERS
9%

DISTRIBUTORS
26%

HOSPITALS
37%

EXPORTS
28%

Fig. 2. Market segmentation of the US medical device industry (2019). (*Adapted from* Curran J. IBISWorld Industry Report 33451b Medical Device Manufacturing in the US. June 2019. Used with permission from IBISWorld Inc.)

The market for low-risk devices such as examination gloves possesses many of these forces, resulting in a highly competitive market. By contrast, the market for high-risk devices lacks these forces, allowing manufacturers to charge higher prices for their products and sustain considerable profits.

Relatively few manufacturers supply the majority of high-risk devices. For example, 5 manufacturers control 90% of the market for hip and knee implants.[8] Furthermore, lack of price transparency limits hospitals from negotiating prices with suppliers. Device manufacturers often require a confidentiality agreement in the purchasing contract with hospitals, which prevents hospitals from disclosing prices to physicians, patients, and insurers.[10] As a result, it becomes difficult to determine price differences among hospitals, a significant setback for price negotiations. It should be noted that there is increasing public demand for price transparency,[11] which may ultimately shift the landscape for negotiation and price setting.

Innovation Trends

Current emphasis on cost reduction while maintaining the quality of patient care has led to new trends in technological innovation. Frugal innovation, which involves creating simpler products with lower unit cost, has become increasingly sought after by the medical device industry.

A subset of frugal innovation, "reverse innovation," specifically has potential in reducing health care expenditure. The phrase refers to developing simpler versions of medical equipment that is already in the market, with the assumption being that these simpler versions will greatly reduce the cost of production and operation.[12] For example, Siemens developed a fetal heart rate monitor that relies on simple microphones as opposed to expensive ultrasound technology that requires specialized training. Not only does this reverse innovation reduce production costs but it also eliminates the added cost of specialized personnel to operate the device. Often, these "reverse innovations" are born out of resource-poor nations.[12] A prime example is the Stanford-JaipurKnee, a $20 high-performance prosthetic knee joint for amputees who are unable to afford more expensive alternatives that currently populate the market.

Deinstitutionalization, or the creation of innovations that reduce high-cost inpatient care, has also emerged in recent years. These innovations are largely centered around remote monitoring of patients.[12] One such innovation, electronic consultations (eConsults), which reduces the need for in-person specialty consultation, proved that high-quality care can be provided to patients at lower cost. Specialties studied include orthopedics, dermatology, endocrinology, and gastroenterology. On average, eConsults were $84 lower per patient per month, with annual savings of more than $578,592 for Medicaid.[13] When used in the right patient population and circumstances, such innovations could become part of mainstream medical practices, and aid in the mission of the Affordable Care Act (ACA) to provide high-quality care at lower cost.

IMPLICATIONS OF COMPARATIVE EFFECTIVENESS RESEARCH

In 2010, the ACA created a new independent entity, the Patient-Centered Outcomes Research Institute, which was tasked with funding and disseminating comparative effectiveness research (CER). CER has been used for many decades before the ACA, although it gained popularity in light of value-driven health care reforms. Currently, CER functions to identify and eliminate care that is no more effective than cheaper alternatives.

Although CER offers many benefits to payers, it also has certain disadvantages. Policies guided by CER will likely lead to better coverage of comparatively effective treatments. However, there will always be a subset of patients that do not respond well to treatments judged favorably by CER. In addition, there will be treatments that do not lend themselves to be rigorously evaluated by CER, such as a lower extremity limb reconstruction and brachial plexus reconstruction, given the vast heterogeneity of clinical presentations. With coverage policies guided by CER, it will be more difficult for these subsets of patients to have access to alternative treatments. Similarly, coverage policies guided by CER could stifle treatment innovations that are only effective in a minor population of patients.[14]

Implementation of CER poses unique challenges. Because CER will be used to guide future policies and influence the types of devices present in the market, it is critical that these studies are adequately designed and interpreted. Potential challenges include the short life cycle of medical devices and relatively short time frame of these studies.

Medical devices have short life cycles because of the incremental changes that are made to devices after entering the market. Such incremental changes are common. For example, the median number of postmarket changes in an orthopedic device's life span is 6.5; 22% of these changes have altered the device design or components.[15] At this rate, devices become substantially different over the years from that which was initially approved, a process known as "design drift."[15]

The rapid rate of change in these devices would make it difficult for CER studies to adjust their study design, resulting in findings that would be based on medical technology that is several generations older than current devices available in the market. Because many of these adjustments can cause significant changes in device safety and efficacy, CER and the policies guided by these studies would not accurately reflect these changes.[16]

In addition, medical devices often require upfront costs, although cost-effectiveness improves over a lifetime. CER studies involving medical devices, however, evaluate patient outcomes over relatively short periods of time, so full clinical benefit may not be observed during this time frame. This must be taken into consideration when evaluating medical devices against other therapies. For example, the cost-effectiveness of implantable cardioverter-defibrillator therapies can range from about $150,000 to $300,000 at 3 years, but drops substantially to about $50,000 to $100,000 over a lifetime.[17]

CER provides a systematic approach to evaluating the efficacy of medical devices. In the future, policies driven by CER must consider the beneficial and harmful effects that CER may have on market diversity. Furthermore, limitations of CER arising from short device life cycles and methodologic shortcomings must also be considered.

REFORMS IN DEVICE APPROVAL AND SURVEILLANCE

The FDA categorizes medical devices into 3 classes, class I, class II, or class III, based on the risk they pose to patients (**Table 3**). Devices that pose greater risk are subject to more regulatory controls and are required to provide evidence of safety and efficacy. Class I, or low-risk devices such as gloves and routine surgical equipment, generally do not require FDA review before they are marketed. On the other hand, class II devices require 510(k) notification, whereby the device must demonstrate that it is "substantially equivalent" to another device in the market.[18] Lastly, class III devices, such as heart valves and orthopedic implants, must submit a premarket approval application, which requires clinical data demonstrating safety and efficacy of the device.[2]

Premarket Approval

The premarket approval process has in recent years drawn criticism for allowing high-risk devices to pass into the market without robust clinical data. It has also been criticized for approving changes to high-risk devices already existing in the market. This process consists of filing "supplements," which tend to have short review times and require minimal supporting data. The number of supplements that can be submitted per device is unlimited. Hence, a device can undergo a series of changes resulting in a version that is substantially different from the initial premarket approval. Such was the case for a femoral component of a hip replacement device that was found to fracture prematurely on the left side when the location of the etched icon of the company was changed to the left side.[16] The ability of manufacturers to make design changes to high-risk devices without adequate oversight and supporting clinical data poses a significant safety concern to patients.

The 510(k) notification process has been the main focus of recent premarket approval reform efforts. The 510(k) requires devices to be "substantially equivalent" to those in the market, and was enacted as a part of the 1976 Federal Food, Drug, and Cosmetic Act.[19] The process requires manufacturers to prove equivalence to a device that is already in the market, known as a predicate device, of their own choosing. Many of these predicate devices were cleared through the 510(k) with preamendment devices serving as predicate devices. In effect, devices are being compared with preamendment safety standards, when there were no requirements for manufacturers to provide clinical evidence. Furthermore, the criteria used to approve a device as "substantially equivalent" is unclear and inconsistent. The process also lacks transparency, preventing physicians and patients from educating themselves about the devices they are using.[20] Therefore, "substantially equivalent" does not necessarily indicate that a product is safe or efficacious.

The DePuy ASR XL Acetabular System for total hip arthroplasty provides an example of the flaws of the 510(k) notification. In 2005, the ASR was cleared by the FDA under the grounds of being "substantially equivalent" to existing implants. Following market entry, it was found that 21% of these implants had to be revised within 4 years.[21] In reviewing the case, it was brought to light that the ASR, although a class III device, was able to be approved through the 510(k) as opposed to the lengthier premarket approval process.[21] Furthermore, the predicate device used for 510(k) approval was significantly different in design from the ASR. The ASR is a "metal-on-metal" type of articulation between components of the hip replacement, whereas the predicate devices are largely "metal-on-plastic."[22]

Table 3
FDA classification of medical devices

Category	Examples	Approval Requirements
Class I (low risk)	• Examination gloves • Compression device • Bone tamp	Registration only
Class II (moderate risk)	• Infusion pumps • Open reduction internal fixation plates • Intramedullary nails	510(k) notification
Class III (high risk)	• Heart valves • Total disc replacements • Mobile-bearing total knee arthroplasty systems	Premarket approval application

Adapted from The Medicare Payment Advisory Commission (MedPAC). An overview of the medical device industry. Report to the Congress: Medicare and the Health Care Delivery System. Washington, D.C.: 2017; with permission.

Although some are urging the FDA to require more clinical data before allowing market entrance, the medical device industry has concerns over increased regulation on time to market and its potential to stunt innovation. The FDA has since been tasked with balancing the concern for premature market entrance with potential delay in time to market. Recently, the FDA has taken steps to strengthen 510(k). Among these efforts are: (1) Eliminating the use of 510(k) for class III devices. Between 2003 and 2009, there were on average 80 submissions for class III devices cleared through 510(k). In 2018, this was brought down to zero.[23] (2) Use of newer predicates. Previously, 20% of 510(k) were cleared based on predicates that were greater than 10 years old. To more closely reflect modern technology, the FDA plans to develop proposals to "sunset" older predicates. (3) Establishment of an alternative 510(k) pathway, the "Safety and Performance Pathway," which would provide manufacturers with objective safety and performance criteria recognized by the FDA as substantial equivalence. This would in turn create transparency for payers who are looking to compare similar devices in the market.[23]

Postmarket Surveillance

As a part of premarket approval, medical devices often undergo studies that are small-scale and in limited patient populations. Following approval, these products are used in a highly diverse patient population and over extended periods of time. Accordingly, it is critical that these devices continue to be monitored for safety and efficacy in these new settings through postmarket surveillance.

Postmarket surveillance methods can be broadly classified as passive and active.[24] Medical device reporting (MDR) remains at the core of the FDA's passive surveillance methods. Medical device–related adverse events can be reported through MDR by manufacturers, physicians, and patients. The FDA, however, has been criticized for delayed and inconsistent response to these reports. Furthermore, many of the reports were missing critical information regarding the adverse event and device identification. This has in turn made it difficult to tease out device malfunction from procedural and user errors.[20,24] The combination of inadequate reporting to FDA and inconsistent FDA response has led to a broken and outdated system for monitoring the increasingly complex and high-risk medical devices being approved today.

Active surveillance consists of clinical studies and medical product registries that collect safety and performance data. The FDA can mandate studies under 2 provisions, postapproval and 522 studies. Postapproval studies can be ordered alongside a premarket approval application, whereas 522 studies can be mandated at any time during a device's life cycle. The postapproval registry surveillance is another form of active surveillance, which can provide long-term safety information unable to be provided by short-term trials.[24]

In recent years, medical device recalls have led to concerns regarding the FDA's postmarket surveillance methods. Aware of these shortcomings, the FDA responded to these concerns with a series of reforms beginning in 2012.[18] Together these reforms aimed to create a systematic method of collecting and analyzing medical device performance data. The first of these reforms was establishing the unique device identification (UDI) system. UDI provides standardization in documenting devices. As a result, the investigation of adverse event reports can be conducted in a timely manner. It also aids in effectively organizing recalls.[25]

The second main reform was the development of the National Evaluation System for health Technology (NEST). NEST received seed funding in 2016 and has since been run by the nonprofit Medical Device Innovation Consortium.[26] Through NEST, the FDA will gain access to multiple sources of electronic health data including insurance claims and medical device performance. With systematic long-term data collection, NEST can facilitate device evaluation across a large patient population and also help identify potential safety concerns sooner.[18]

MEDICAL DEVICE EXCISE TAX

In 2013, the ACA imposed a 2.3% excise tax on medical devices, one of many provisions that served as a revenue source for health care reform. It was projected to collect $29 billion of net revenues over 10 years. Since the introduction of this tax, there has been a large debate surrounding the potential harm it may pose to research and development in medical device companies. In light of this controversy, a 2-year moratorium was imposed on the tax.[27]

Opponents of the medical device tax claim that it will reduce R&D spending by approximately 20%. In recent years, R&D investment has been declining (15.5% in 2000–2007 to 4.7% in 2013–2017[28]). Although this is likely multifactorial, opponents are concerned that implementing the tax would lead to an even higher reduction in R&D expenses. The tax would also have a negative impact on small and startup companies because it is based on a fixed percentage of sales, and these companies do not typically achieve profitability until their annual sales exceeds $100 million to $150 million. Because small companies are a major source of innovation, this could likely stunt development of new technologies.[9,27]

Proponents of the tax claim that it serves as a revenue source for financial health reform, and it would be difficult to find alternative sources. Furthermore, the tax will offset increased profitability for medical devices as a result of health care expansion.[3]

In early 2019, a bipartisan bill known as the Protect Medical Innovation Act of 2019 was introduced in both the House of Representatives and Senate. This bill would permanently repeal the medical device excise tax effective as of 2020.

SUMMARY

The medical device industry has withstood many changes as a result of value-based health care reforms. These reforms have affected device development at various stages, mainly funding for prototyping and the market approval process. Increased regulations surrounding premarket approval and postmarket surveillance have improved the safety of devices entering the market, accompanied however by a likely increased time to market, an unfavorable effect for entrepreneurs and manufacturers alike. In addition, the introduction of new payment models has driven the creation of cost efficient innovations. However, market dynamics continue to be difficult to change because of the lack of price transparency and control of the market by a small number of sellers. Lastly, CER serves as a useful tool for creating value-based coverage policies. To promote health care equity, policy makers must take into consideration the impact of CER on accessibility of alternative treatments for patient subgroups.

DISCLOSURE

NIH NIAMS grant K23AR073928.

REFERENCES

1. Curran J. IBISWorld industry report 33451b. Medical device manufacturing in the US. IBISWorld; 2019.
2. MedPac. Report to the Congress: Medicare and the health care delivery system. An overview of the medical device industry. Available at: http://www.medpac.gov/docs/default-source/reports/jun17_reporttocongress_sec.pdf. Accessed June, 2017.
3. Congressional Research Service. The medical device excise tax: economic analysis. Available at: https://fas.org/sgp/crs/misc/R43342.pdf. Accessed June, 2015.
4. Donahoe G, King G. Estimates of medical device spending in the United States. Advanced Medical Technology Association. Available at: https://www.advamed.org/sites/default/files/resource/994_100515_guy_king_report_2015_final.pdf. Accessed June, 2015.
5. Panescu D. Medical device development. 2009 Annual International Conference of the IEEE Engineering in Medicine and Biology Society. Minneapolis (MN): Institute of Electrical and Electronics Engineers; 2009. p. 5591–4.
6. Innovation Counselors LLC. A future at risk: economic performance, entrepreneurship, and venture capital in the U.S. medical technology sector. Washington (DC): AdvaMed; 2016.
7. Fleming JJ. The decline of venture capital investment in early-stage life sciences poses a challenge to continued innovation. Health Aff 2015;34(2):271–6.
8. Lind K. Understanding the market for implantable medical devices. AARP Public Policy Institute. Insight on the Issues 2017;129:1–15.
9. Nexon D, Ubl SJ. Implications of health reform for the medical technology industry. Health Aff 2010; 29(7):1325–9.
10. Robinson J, Bridy A. Confidentiality and transparency for medical device prices: market dynamics and policy alternatives. Berkeley center for health technology. Available at: https://bcht.berkeley.edu/sites/default/files/device-prices-transparency-report.pdf. Accessed October, 2009.
11. Wilensky G. Federal government increases focus on price transparency. JAMA 2019;322(10):916.
12. Mattke S, Liu H, Orr P. Medical device innovation in the era of the affordable care act: the end of sexy. Rand Health Q 2016;6(1):9.
13. Anderson D, Villagra VG, Coman E, et al. Reduced cost of specialty care using electronic consultations for Medicaid patients. Health Aff 2018;37(12): 2031–6.
14. Basu A, Jena AB, Philipson TJ. The impact of comparative effectiveness research on health and health care spending. J Health Econ 2011;30(4): 695–706.
15. Samuel AM, Rathi VK, Grauer JN, et al. How do orthopaedic devices change after their initial FDA premarket approval? Clin Orthop Relat Research 2016;474(4):1053–68.
16. Jalbert JJ, Ritchey ME, Mi X, et al. Methodological considerations in observational comparative effectiveness research for implantable medical devices: an epidemiologic perspective. Am J Epidemiol 2014;180(9):949–58.
17. Sharma A, Blank A, Patel P, et al. Health care policy and regulatory implications on medical device innovations: a cardiac rhythm medical device industry

perspective. J Interv Card Electrophysiol 2013; 36(2):107–17.

18. Medical device safety action plan: protecting patients, promoting public health. Washington (DC): FDA; 2018.

19. Wizemann T. Public health effectiveness of the FDA 510(k) clearance process: balancing patient safety and innovation: workshop report. Washington (DC): National Academies Press; 2010.

20. Fargen KM, Frei D, Fiorella D, et al. The FDA approval process for medical devices: an inherently flawed system or a valuable pathway for innovation? J Neurointerv Surg 2013;5(4):269–75.

21. Curfman GD, Redberg RF. Medical devices—balancing regulation and innovation. N Engl J Med 2011;365(11):975–7.

22. Cohen D. Out of joint: the story of the ASR. BMJ 2011;342(may13 2):d2905.

23. FDA has taken steps to strengthen the 510(k) program. Washington (DC): FDA; 2018.

24. Rajan PV, Kramer DB, Kesselheim AS. Medical device postapproval safety monitoring: where does the United States stand? Circ Cardiovasc Qual Outcomes 2015;8(1):124–31.

25. Daniel G, Colvin H, Khaterzai S, et al. Strengthening patient care: building an effective national medical device surveillance system. Washington (DC): The Brookings Institution; 2015.

26. National evaluation system for health technology (NEST). Washington (DC): FDA; 2019.

27. Lee D. Impact of the excise tax on firm R&D and performance in the medical device industry: evidence from the affordable care act. Res Policy 2018; 47(5):854–71.

28. Pulse of the industry: EY medical technology report 2017. EY; 2017.

Health Policy in Hand Surgery
Evaluating What Works

Lauren M. Shapiro, MD[a], Robin N. Kamal, MD[b],*

KEYWORDS

- Bundled care • Hand surgery • Health policy • Patient outcomes • Quality evaluation

KEY POINTS

- The Patient Protection and Affordable Care Act, signed into law in 2010 to address the unsustainable rate of growth in health care costs of the US health care system, introduced complex provisions that affect hand surgeons.
- Alternative payment models, such as bundled payments, have been introduced and show promise for some orthopedic episodes of care. Although not yet applied to hand surgery, understanding the strengths and weaknesses of these programs can inform efforts to implement bundled payments in hand surgery.
- Although rigorous investigation on the development and implementation of predictive models and outcome measures (specifically patient-reported outcome measures) has been completed, assessment of their effectiveness in improving patient care, and in alternative payment models is lacking.

INTRODUCTION

Health policy is a broad topic, but an integral aspect of our medical specialty that not only drives decisions and actions of hand surgeons but also directly affects patient care. Therefore, it is important to understand what policies exist and how they affect the practice of hand surgery now, and how they may affect the specialty in the future. A critical analysis of new initiatives and payment models, and their clinical effectiveness on patient outcomes, can shape future investigations and care delivery models focused on improving patient health.

The Basics

When assessing health policy and health care reform, it is important to critically evaluate 3 key dimensions:

1. The specificity of the policy
2. The stakeholders affected
3. The evaluation framework being used

Details of the specific populations, timelines, and so forth, allow for an evaluation of the process for implementation, barriers (eg, cultural) and expected outcomes of the policy. For example, a policy that advocates for "increasing access to timely care" lacks specificity to the population and measurement criteria and therefore does not allow for appropriate evaluation. A better example may include a target population (eg, all patients below the poverty line) and specifics about how to define timely care (eg, undergoing reduction of a dislocated joint within 6 hours). Understanding the stakeholders involved and a policy's implications on each is fundamental in evaluating the expected outcomes of a policy in addition to

[a] Department of Orthopaedic Surgery, Stanford University, 300 Pasteur Drive, Room R1444, Mail Code: 5341, Stanford, CA 94305, USA; [b] Department of Orthopaedic Surgery, Stanford University, 450 Broadway Street MC: 6342, Redwood City, CA 94603, USA
* Corresponding author.
E-mail address: rnkamal@stanford.edu

Hand Clin 36 (2020) 263–270
https://doi.org/10.1016/j.hcl.2020.01.009
0749-0712/20/© 2020 Elsevier Inc. All rights reserved.

unintended consequences. Key stakeholders to consider include the patient, the physician, family members and caretakers, the payor, society, and the policymaker. Stakeholders may have competing interests and/or different viewpoints on policies and their effectiveness. For example, when evaluating the cost of a particular policy or reform, the cost to the patient (eg, missing time from work) and the payor (eg, direct costs and downstream costs) may be vastly different. Finally, having a clear framework and outcome measures to characterize and understand the effectiveness of a policy is critical to ensure expected outcomes are indeed realized, unintended consequences are minimized, and opportunities for improvement are maximized.

Current Environment

In 2015 the Medicare Access and CHIP Reauthorization Act (MACRA) was signed into law.[1] The Quality Payment Program (QPP) was instituted under MACRA and is established on a system based on quality of care, and the cost to deliver care (value) in lieu of the fee-for-service model. This shift from fee-for-service (a system that rewards the delivery of more services without measuring quality) to a value-based reimbursement system, where quality and cost are explicitly defined and measured, aims to decrease the unsustainable cost of the US health care system.[2] The Merit-based Incentive Payment System (MIPS) is 1 method of participation in the QPP that determines Medicare payment adjustments. MIPS is comprised of 4 components:

1. Medicare Electronic Health Records
2. Physician Quality Reporting System
3. Value-based Payment Modifier
4. Improvement Activities

Value-based care places increased responsibility and risk on health care organizations to continuously improve quality of care while decreasing the overall cost of care compared with benchmarks.

Registries

The ability to measure and evaluate outcomes is fundamental to the implementation of value-based care. Some provisions of the Patient Protection and Affordable Care Act (ACA) foster the creation of registries with the vision that standardized data collection increases accountability and transparency while allowing for insights into outcomes, complications, and value in care delivery. Registries have historically been used for implant surveillance; however, registries have recently been developed that focus on collecting outcomes from the patient perspective (eg, patient-reported outcome measures [PROMs]), such as the American Joint Replacement Registry and the Function and Outcomes Research for Comparative Effectiveness in Total Joint Replacement. Although few registries for hand surgery exist, examples include the national quality registry for hand surgery (HAKIR [Handkirurgiskt kvalitetsregister]) in Sweden[3] and from the Congenital Upper Limb Differences (CoULD) registry.[4,5]

Although registries present several challenges (eg, cost, lack of standardized outcome measures, loss to follow-up, variation in important data elements for conditions), they allow for many benefits, including longitudinal tracking of outcomes, comparison across surgeons and organizations, more accurate risk adjustment, which all have the potential to contribute to and improve value. The HAKIR project began in 2010 and has expanded to include all 7 hand surgery departments in Sweden by 5 years.[3] In 5 years, the HAKIR project collected data on almost 60,000 hand surgery procedures. The CoULD registry was implemented in 2014 by 2 pediatric hand centers and has expanded to include multiple centers around the United States.[4,5] In 2 years, they enrolled more than 500 children with congenital upper limb differences and were able to collect robust demographic, clinical, and radiographic data. Hand surgery currently lacks a comprehensive, prospective data registry system. Although there are multiple logistical and scientific challenges to prospective data collection in a hand surgery registry, the implementation of such a registry would ideally integrate across several electronic medical records, have low administrative and input burden (to office staff and patients), allow for real-time data analysis, which is important for clinical decision making, and clearly define outcome measures important to patients and surgeons for each clinical condition.

Bundled Care

Bundled care models are a form of an alternative payment model that aim to deliver greater value during an episode of care for a given condition (eg, 90 days after total joint arthroplasty). In a bundled care model, an episode of care is defined for a condition or a medical event during a defined period of time and a lump-sum payment is provided to the facility per episode of care. Although this requires health systems to assume some risk (eg, they are responsible for the excess cost if the cost of the care provided goes above the lump-sum payment), they may also share in the upside (eg, they share in the savings if costs are kept below the lump-sum price if quality is not compromised). Bundled care models incentivize physicians to enhance care coordination and efficiency to improve quality while decreasing cost. These models, however, have limitations in accurate risk adjustment, continuing to incentivize operative treatment, and competition toward decreasing costs without clearly defining quality of care from the patient perspective.

Medicare introduced a mandatory bundled care payment model, Comprehensive Care for Joint Replacement (CJR), for in-patient hip and knee replacement in 2016 in select areas. The initiation of CJR is a unique analytical opportunity as CJR randomly mandated metropolitan statistical areas (MSAs) to participate.[6,7] Barnett and colleagues[8] conducted a difference-in-difference analysis of Medicare claims data encompassing the first 2 years of bundled care for CJR and evaluated before and after implementation of 75 MSAs that were randomly mandated to participate and 121 control MSAs. Adjusting for hospital and patient characteristics and procedures, they demonstrated greater decreases in institutional spending per episode of care in the bundled care payment MSAs as compared with the control MSAs, which was largely driven by a decrease in patients discharged to post-acute care facilities. Importantly, there were no differences noted in complication rates or in patients selected (as measured by percentage of "high-risk" patients included). Encouraging is that the decrease this group noted in payments increased over an 18-month period, raising the possibility that reductions in payments (and possibly improvement in value) may continue to expand as hospitals and systems adapt to the new model. However, bundled payments are limited by a lack of incorporation of patient-centered outcomes as a measure of quality. There are also concerns that financial incentives will be prioritized over patient outcomes to achieve less costly care.

In hand surgery, early survey studies of the American Society for Surgery of the Hand members demonstrated that about 68% of respondents disagreed or strongly disagreed that the ACA would improve health care in the United States and that 37% believed that implementation would cause them to retire earlier than anticipated.[9] Despite this outlook, these survey respondents admitted to having little knowledge of the law. Although there are no currently mandated bundles in hand surgery, bundled care payment models for hand surgical care may be developed and it is essential for hand surgeons to understand their mechanics to inform strategies to achieve success in these payment models.

In anticipation of a bundled care payment model, investigators have begun to not only examine costs of care associated with distal radius fractures, but also to develop bundled payment schemes and evaluate the implications of various definitions of episodes of care.[10] Other investigators have evaluated the effect of identifying and removing cost drivers that do not lead to improved quality of care.[11] By identifying areas of opportunity and incorporating changes in processes of care (eg, evidence-based protocols for wide-awake local anesthesia, education with surgical staff), the authors were able to demonstrate a 31% reduction in total direct costs, significant decreases in various time measures (eg, total patient time in the facility, PACU to discharge time) with no change in quality. Similar methodology (creation and review of current state process map to identify areas of high variation, costs, and/or opportunity, systematic review of quality measures and/or high-value evidence-based implementation changes, application of the above measures/changes, and reevaluation) can be applied to various episodes of care not only in anticipation of bundled care models in the future but for the provision of high-quality care for current patients.

Predictive Modeling

Although many organizations have demonstrated success in the implementation of bundled care payment models for hip and knee replacement,[12–14] the external validity of these models comes into question when evaluating other conditions or when attempting to appropriately account for patient-specific risk factors. As an example, given the success of the bundled care payment models in hip and knee replacement, a proposal was set forth in 2016 to extend the bundled episode of care to hip fractures.[15] Grace and colleagues,[16] reported on the experience of 1 institution with bundled care payment models and the differences in costs incurred by performing a total hip replacement for hip arthritis as compared with a femoral neck fracture. In reference to the target price (the money allocated for each episode of care), total hip arthroplasty for a femoral neck fracture resulted in a loss of $415,950 as compared with a gain of $172,448 for hip arthritis. This discrepancy is likely due at least in part to the fact that those patients undergoing a total hip arthroplasty for a hip fracture (as compared with those undergoing a total hip arthroplasty for arthritis) are older, have more comorbidities, and cannot be equally optimized compared with elective surgery, increasing their risk of complications and associated costs.[17,18] This highlights the importance of risk adjustment and the nuances in applying bundled care payment models for various conditions, populations, and geographic locations.

Evolving technologies may assist in creating improved models. Machine learning has been recently applied to medical decision making and may serve to advance value-based care models by improving risk stratification based on patient demographic and other factors that affect length of stay and risk of complications.[19–21] To investigate this, Karnuta and colleagues,[15] developed a Naive Bayes machine-learning algorithm for patients who had undergone surgery for hip fracture with preoperative patient data to predict length of stay and associated costs. Although their model demonstrated accuracies of 77% and 79% for length of stay and cost, respectively, and demonstrated 88% and 89% performance for length of stay and cost, respectively, they most importantly demonstrated that costs associated with hip fracture care are primarily nonmodifiable patient-specific factors, raising concerns for the application of bundled care payment models for this condition. Even though elective management of hip arthritis allows for medical optimization and preoperative planning, the value-based incentivization of bundled care payment models may not be best suited for conditions in which outcomes or cost are primarily driven by nonmodifiable patient-level elements.

Electronic health predictive analysis is growing rapidly (primarily on the premise that these predictive models can forecast whether or not a patient will experience a complication of a specific treatment or if procedure A is likely to benefit a patient more so than compared with procedure B), but very little consideration has been paid to the effect of these models on patient outcomes or the accuracy and validity of such models.[22,23] For example, no model coefficients or accuracy data were originally reported for the American Joint Replacement Registry risk calculator that is frequently used to estimate 90-day mortality risk and 2-year prosthetic joint infection risk for total joint replacement.[24] Several recent studies have shown the external validity of various calculators and models having poor accuracy[25–27] and limited application at the time needed (eg, cannot be used preoperatively as the model includes characteristics obtained during the hospital stay).[26,28,29]

Harris[22] described a practical framework to guide use, evaluation, and implementation of surgical predictive models with a focus on improving patient outcomes. The author suggests that predictive models should:

1. Include important and modifiable outcomes
2. Include inputs that will be available at the time of decision
3. Be accurate given the clinical context

4. Be cross-validated using data not used in the development of the model
5. Be useable and accessible in a technology platform

Standards set forth in the Transparent Reporting of a Multivariable Prediction Model for Individual Prognosis or Diagnosis and the recent consensus statement further reiterate many of these themes.[30,31] The framework described includes 6 conditions that should be met to ensure predictive models create value and benefit patients.

Outcome Measures

Evaluating value and the implementation of registries, bundled care payment models, and predictive models requires an understanding of how value and its components are defined and measured. Generally speaking, value is defined as the quality of care delivered by the cost; however, there are several nuances associated with this definition. Definitions of quality are typically defined within the context of the Donabedian model[32] of structure, process, and outcomes. Similar to the definition of value, defining quality is also equally nuanced. PROMs are instruments designed to capture a patient's health status, specific symptoms, or quality of life (as opposed to other more objective and nonpatient defined measures, such as range of motion or complication rate). Four critical aspects to consider when evaluating value and outcomes include that these definitions and measurements:

1. Are traditionally aimed toward health care delivery for a population as a whole
2. May vary significantly by stakeholder
3. May not account for the appropriateness of care
4. And may vary by the context in which they are applied

Although many organizations are collecting PROMs before and after surgery, these data have historically been collected to understand outcomes at a health system or population level, not at the individual patient level, or to inform individual patient decision making. For example, although tools (eg, decision aids) to educate and aid patients in decision making aligned with their values and preferences have been advocated by several organizations[33,34] and have demonstrated positive effects on patient knowledge, communication, expectations, and so forth,[35–37] their role is not fully maximized when they are not individualized to a specific patient and instead rely on average, population risk information. For example, preliminary work by Bansback and colleagues[38] and Gutacker and Street[39] demonstrated that information provided on decision aids lacked salience and validity because individual patients feel they are not only different but have varying expectations from the "average" patient. Additional qualitative work has demonstrated that many goals defined by patients are not queried on standardized PROMs in surgery (eg, yoga, hiking).[40] It is becoming more evident that decision-making tools and outcome measures may be even more powerful when combined with measures tailored to the individual patient.

The collection of PROMs serves to benefit all stakeholders, but each stakeholder has his/her own goals and value proposition. Franklin and colleagues[41] laid out a framework and aimed to identify the value of PROMs by stakeholder. The 4 defined subsets of PROM users include:

1. Patients and physicians
2. Hospital leaders and clinicians
3. Insurers and hospital leaders
4. Researchers, policy makers, and funders

Although the goals and values of PROM use by stakeholder groups are not mutually exclusive, having an understanding of each stakeholder's perspective and what each stands to gain from a specific measurement parameter is important (eg, outcome as measured by cost and usefulness may be critical to insurers, but the cost of care may be less important to patients and physicians).

Appropriate use criteria (AUC) specify when it is appropriate to perform a medical procedure based on evidence or, in the absence of evidence, expert consensus. AUC may be helpful in guiding medical decision making; however, it is important to note that many AUC do not incorporate PROMs (or patient-specific health-related quality of life factors), nor do excellent posttreatment PROMs ensure appropriate care. For example, the American Academy of Orthopaedic Surgeons AUC for the treatment of distal radius fractures incorporates fracture type, mechanism of injury, activity level of patient, patient health, and associated injuries, but does not account for the level of symptoms. Similarly, an elderly, infirm patient with low functional demands treated operatively for a proximal humerus fracture who reports excellent PROM scores postoperatively may not denote appropriate use. The incorporation of AUC into PROMs and vice versa may promote a more quantifiable patient-centered approach to decision making.

Finally, a growing body of research has demonstrated that factors (both modifiable and nonmodifiable) and the context in which PROMs are administered may influence scores.[42–47] In reviewing psychosocial factors affecting PROMs of adults sustaining an isolated elbow fracture, Jayakumar and colleagues[47] demonstrated kinesiophobia and self-efficacy to be strong predictors of postinjury limitation. Multiple investigators have reported the impact of depression and other psychosocial metrics on orthopedic PROMs.[43–45,47] Furthermore, other investigators have demonstrated that varying the context in which PROMs are administered (having patients complete functional tasks before PROM administration as compared with patients not completing functional tasks before PROM administration) has an impact on PROM scores above minimal clinically important differences.[46] It is critical that future work further elucidates these effects to add further granularity to processes that strive to improve the value of care provided.

Hospital Ratings and Rankings

In an effort to evaluate hospital quality and performance, several rating systems have been developed that are used in various ways, including allowing patients to decide where to receive care, identifying areas for improvement, and establishing contracts with high performing centers. In highly competitive markets, hospitals may have much to gain and/or a lot to lose based on these ratings. Although transparency is important to provide patients and health systems alike with information regarding health system performance, misclassification and a lack of reliability or validity are major concerns. It is unknown how many patients use hospital ranking systems to evaluate providers or how much revenue is brought into a system by such rankings. The fact that lawsuits have been brought in response to certain ratings further emphasizes the importance of understanding the composition and implications of the ratings.[48]

Billamora and colleagues[49] recently conducted an evaluation and comparison of major US publicly reported hospital quality rating systems (eg, US News & World Reports, Leapfrog Safety Grade, and Top Hospitals) through expert analysis of the literature and in discussion with leaders from each rating system. Using 6 evaluation criteria of:

1. Potential for misclassification of hospital performance
2. Importance/impact
3. Scientific acceptability
4. Iterative improvement
5. Transparency
6. Usability

They concluded that, on an A scale (an ideal rating system with little change of misclassifying hospital performance) to F scale (a poor rating system that is more likely to misclassify performance than to assign it correctly), no rating system earned higher than a B, with the lowest groups receiving a D+. Common shortcomings of several rating systems included the data measurement limitations (eg, use of administrative data, which are designed for billing, is less granular, and has been shown to have a high false-positive and false-negative rates), lack of a robust data auditing system (eg, to ensure accurate data reporting), and potential financial conflicts (eg, having hospitals pay rating systems to use their ratings for marketing), to name a few.

There are many features highlighted here in evaluating rating systems that are similarly shortcomings in the evaluation of quality itself. Many of these include acquiring clinically meaningful data that are reliable and valuable to many stakeholders, allowing for adequate risk adjustment, and having a demonstrated association with patient outcomes. A complete understanding of the shortcomings of not only rating systems but the evaluation of quality and policy in health care can guide future health policy strategy in hand surgery.

SUMMARY

Much is changing with regard to current health care policy and its influence on the hand surgical landscape. Because these policies are complicated and nuanced, much investigation is required to implement these policies properly to ensure high-quality care delivery for patients. Although many policies are broadly applied, it is critical to use caution and have a thorough understanding of the potential implications before widespread approval.

DISCLOSURE

RNK: National Institutes of Health award (K23AR073307-01).

REFERENCES

1. MACRA: MIPS, APMs. Centers for Medicare & Medicaid Services. Available at: https://www.cms.gov/Medicare/Quality-Initiatives-Patient-Assessment-Instruments/Value-Based-Programs/MACRA-MIPS-and-APMs/MACRA-MIPS-and-APMs.html. Accessed August 9, 2019.
2. Laugesen MJ, Glied SA. Higher fees paid to US physicians drive higher spending for physician services compared to other countries. Health Aff (Millwood) 2011;30(9):1647–56.
3. Arner M. Developing a national quality registry for hand surgery: challenges and opportunities. EFFORT Open Rev 2016;1:100–6.
4. Vuillermin C, Canizares MF, Bauer AS, et al. Congenital upper limb differences registry: development and challenges of a prospective database. J Hand Surg Am 2017;42:s21–2.
5. Bae DS, Canizares MF, Miller PE, et al. Functional impact of congenital hand differences: early results from the Congenital Upper Limb Differences (CoULD) registry. J Hand Surg Am 2018;43:321–30.
6. Mechanic RE. Mandatory Medicare bundled payment—is it ready for prime time? N Engl J Med 2015;373:1291–3.
7. Wadhera RK, Yeh RW, Joynt Maddox KE. The rise and fall of mandatory cardiac bundled payments. JAMA 2018;319:335–6.
8. Barnett ML, Wilcock A, Michael McWilliams J, et al. Two-year evaluation of mandatory bundled payments for joint replacement. N Engl J Med 2019; 380:252–62.
9. Shubinets V, Gerety PA, Pannucci CJ, et al. Attitude of hand surgeons toward Affordable Care Act: a survey of members of the American Society for Surgery of the Hand. J Orthop 2016;14:38–44.
10. Jubelt LE, Goldfeld KS, Blecker SB, et al. Early lessons on bundled payment at an academic medical center. J Am Acad Orthop Surg 2017;25:654–63.
11. Huetteman HE, Zhong L, Chung KC. Cost of surgical treatment for distal radius fractures and the implications of episode-based bundled payments. J Hand Surg Am 2018;43:720–30.
12. Kamal RN, Behal R. Clinical care redesign to improve value in carpal tunnel syndrome: a before and after implementation study. J Hand Surg Am 2019;44:1–8.
13. Edwards PK, Mears SC, Barnes CL. BPCI: everyone wins, including the patient. J Arthroplasty 2017;32: 1728–31.
14. Courtney PM, Ashley BS, Hume EL, et al. Are bundled payments a viable reimbursement model for revision total joint arthroplasty? Clin Orthop Relat Res 2016;474:2714–21.
15. Karnuta JM, Navarro SM, Baeberle HS, et al. Bundled care for hip fractures: a machine learning approach to an untenable patient-specific payment model. J Orthop Trauma 2019;33:324–30.
16. Grace TR, Patterson JT, Tangtiphaiboontana J, et al. Hip fractures and the bundle: a cost analysis of patients undergoing hip arthroplasty for femoral neck fracture vs degenerative joint disease. J Arthroplasty 2018;33:1681–5.
17. Kester BS, Williams J, Bosco JA, et al. The association between hospital length of stay and 90-day readmission risk for femoral neck patients: within a total joint arthroplasty bundled payment initiative. J Arthroplasty 2016;31:2741–5.

18. Yoon RS, Mahure SA, Hutzler LH, et al. Hip arthroplasty for fracture vs. elective care: one bundle does not fit all. J Arthroplasty 2017;32:2353–8.

19. Beam AL, Kohane IS. Big data and machine learning in health care. JAMA 2018;319:1317.

20. Chen JH, Asch SM. Machine learning and prediction in medicine—beyond the peak of inflated expectations. N Engl J Med 2017;376:2507–9.

21. Delahanty RJ, Kaufman D, Jones SS. Development and evaluation of an automated machine learning algorithm for in-hospital mortality risk adjustment among critical care patients. Crit Care Med 2018;46:1.

22. Harris AHS. Path from predictive analytics to improved patient outcomes: a framework to guide use, implementation, and evaluation of accurate surgical predictive models. Ann Surg 2017;265:461–3.

23. Harris ASH, Kuo AC, Weng Y, et al. Can machine learning methods produce accurate and easy-to-use prediction models of 30-day complications and mortality after knee or hip arthroplasty? Clin Orthop Relat Res 2019;477:452–60.

24. Bozic KJ, Lau E, Kurtz S, et al. Patient-related risk factors for periprosthetic joint infection and postoperative mortality following total hip arthroplasty in Medicare patients. J Bone Joint Surg Am 2012;94:794–800.

25. Harris AHS, Kuo AC, Bozic KJ, et al. American Joint Replacement Registry risk calculator does not predict 90-day mortality in veterans undergoing total joint replacement. Clin Orthop Relat Res 2018;476:1960–75.

26. Mu Y, Edwards JR, Horan TC, et al. Improving risk-adjusted measures of surgical site infection for the National Healthcare Safety Network. Infect Control Hosp Epidemiol 2011;32:970–86.

27. Romine LB, May RG, Taylor HD, et al. Accuracy and clinical utility of a peri-operative risk calculator for total knee arthroplasty. J Arthroplasty 2013;28:445–8.

28. Berbari EF, Osmon DR, Lahr B, et al. The Mayo prosthetic joint infection risk score: implication for surgical site infection reporting and risk stratification. Infect Control Hosp Epidemiol 2012;33:774–81.

29. Wuerz TH, Kent DM, Malchau H, et al. A nomogram to predict major complications after hip and knee arthroplasty. J Arthroplasty 2014;29:1457–62.

30. Collins GS, Reitsma JB, Altman DG, et al. Transparent reporting of a multivariable prediction model for Individual Prognosis Or Diagnosis (TRIPOD). Ann Intern Med 2015;162:735–6.

31. Amarasingham R, Audet AM, Bates DW, et al. Consensus statement on electronic health predictive analytics: a guiding framework to address challenges. EGEMS (Wash DC) 2016;4:1163.

32. Donabedian A. The quality of care. How can it be assessed? JAMA 1988;260:1743–8.

33. The SHARE approach. Agency for Healthcare Research and Quality. Available at: https://www.ahrq.gov/health-literacy/curriculum-tools/shareddecisionmaking/index.html. Accessed August 9, 2019.

34. Shared decision making: a standard of care for all patients. National Quality Foundation. Available at: qualityforum.org/Publications/2017/10/NQP_Shared_Decision_Making_Action_Brief.aspx. Accessed August 9, 2019.

35. Bozic KJ, Belkora J, Chan V, et al. Shared decision making in patients with osteoarthritis of the hip and knee: results of a randomized controlled trial. J Bone Joint Surg Am 2013;95:1633–9.

36. Stacey D, Hawker G, Dervin G, et al. Decision aid for patients considering total knee arthroplasty with preference report for surgeons: a pilot randomized controlled trial. BMC Musculoskelet Disord 2014;15:54.

37. Arterburn D, Wellman R, Westbrook E, et al. Introducing decision aids at group health was linked to sharply lower hip and knee surgery rates and costs. Health Aff (Millwood) 2012;31:2094–104.

38. Bansback N, Trenaman L, Bryan S, et al. Using routine patient reported outcome measures to enhance patient decision making: a proof of concept study. Qual Life Res 2015;24:109.

39. Gutacker N, Street A. Use of large-scale HRQoL datasets to generate individualised predictions and inform patients about the likely benefit of surgery. Qual Life Res 2017;26:2497–505.

40. Wright HH, O'Brien V, Valdes K, et al. Relationship of the patient-specific functional scale to commonly used clinical measures in hand osteoarthritis. J Hand Ther 2017;30:538–45.

41. Franklin P, Chenok K, Lavalee D, et al. Framework to guide the collection and use of patient-reported outcome measures in the learning healthcare system. EGEMS (Wash DC) 2017;5:17.

42. Claessen MD, Jos JJ, Stoop N, et al. Influence on priming on patient-reported outcome measures: a randomized controlled trial. Psychosomatics 2016;57:47–56.

43. Merrill RK, Zebala LP, Peters C, et al. Impact of depression on patient-reported outcome measures after lumbar spine decompression. Spine (Phila Pa 1976) 2018;43:434–9.

44. London DA, Stepan JG, Boyer MI, et al. The impact of depression and pain catastrophization on initial presentation and treatment outcomes for atraumatic hand conditions. J Bone Joint Surg Am 2014;96:806–14.

45. Vranceanu AM, Jupiter JB, Mudgal CS, et al. Predictors of pain intensity and disability after minor hand surgery. J Hand Surg Am 2010;35:956–60.

46. Shapiro LM, Harris AHS, Eppler SL, et al. Can the QuickDASH PROM be altered by first completing

the tasks on the instrument? Clin Orthop Relat Res 2019;477:2069–70.

47. Jayakumar P, Teunis T, Vranceanu AM, et al. Psychosocial factors affecting variation in patient-reported outcomes after elbow fractures. J Shoulder Elbow Surg 2019;28:1431–40.

48. In the age of consumerism, hospital rating can make or break revenue. Healthcare Finance. Available at: https://www.healthcarefinancenews.com/news/age-consumerism-hospital-ratings-can-make-or-break-revenue. Accessed August 9, 2019.

49. Rating the raters: an evaluation of publicly reported hospital quality rating systems. Available at: https://catalyst.nejm.org/evaluation-hospital-quality-rating-systems/. Accessed August 14, 2019.

Advocacy and the Hand Surgeon: Why and How

Kay Kirkpatrick, MD[a],*, Andrew Gurman, MD[b,1]

KEYWORDS

- Advocacy • Political engagement • Political advocacy • Hand surgery • Politics

KEY POINTS

- Political advocacy is important to hand surgeons at the state and federal level because of the many issues in clinical practice that are affected by government.
- Hand surgeons can participate in advocacy as individuals and through their medical organizations.
- ASSH is in a unique position for advocacy because of the multiple specialties involved in the organization.

This article provides the perspective of two hand surgeons who are also health care leaders on why advocacy matters to hand surgeons and how to accomplish goals in the political arena.

For one of us (A.G.), the initiating event was an impending crisis in medical liability coverage. Insurance was in danger of becoming unaffordable and unobtainable. There was a clear need to get involved, and it seemed that advocacy through the state orthopedic society would limit telling the story to orthopedics, whereas working through the state medical society would allow advocacy on behalf of orthopedics, obstetrics/gynecology, neurosurgery, trauma surgery, and other specialties that would be potentially affected. That effort was largely successful, and it prompted me to continue advocating on other topics. That led to a leadership position, and ultimately to the privilege of serving as president of the American Medical Association (AMA). From that position, I was able to advocate in front of Congress on behalf of our patients and our profession.

For the other author (K.K.), advocacy on behalf of my large orthopedic group consisted of participation in the various organizations that represent doctors and specialists in addition to hiring our own lobbyist at the state level and having doctors develop personal relationships with our legislators. We created group memberships that enrolled all of our doctors in our societies (for a discount) to increase our participation. We always viewed membership in these groups as part of our overhead to protect our business model and represent ourselves and our patients. As a leader, it was clear to me that advocacy is an essential part of survival in our challenging environment. Legislators tend to trust doctors and we still have a lot of credibility as long as we keep the conversation focused on the patient. As I neared retirement, an opportunity to serve in a different way presented when my local Senator resigned to run for Congress. I was asked to consider running because we needed more medical voices at our state Capitol. I took up the challenge and was elected to our state Senate in 2017. Since that time, I have authored or cosponsored and passed good health care legislation and have become a go-to person on health care in our legislature.

Although we have worked in different arenas, we are clear on the value of members of our profession taking ownership of issues important to patients and advocating for them at all levels of the political process. Here are some current issues that affect hand surgeons where advocacy can play a role in the conversation.

Federal issues affecting hand surgeons:
1. Surprise billing occurs when a patient goes to a facility for treatment where some of the care providers are not in their insurance

a Georgia State Senate, Atlanta, GA, USA; b Solo Hand Surgery Practice, Altoona, PA, USA
1 Present address: 1701 12th Avenue, Suite C2, Altoona, PA 16601.
* Corresponding author. 324 Coverdell Legislative Office Building, 18 Capitol Square SW, Atlanta, GA 30334.
E-mail address: kaykirkpatrickmd@gmail.com

Hand Clin 36 (2020) 271–274
https://doi.org/10.1016/j.hcl.2020.01.010
0749-0712/20/© 2020 Elsevier Inc. All rights reserved.

network. Because the patient assumes that if the facility is in network the doctors are also, there may be a "surprise" bill that arrives long after the care. There is currently no consistent mechanism for resolving these bills and the patients are in the middle. There are competing federal bills on the subject and it is not yet clear which solution will be advanced. Doctors do not want to be forced to accept a contract they view as unfair. Insurance companies want to set the price at a level acceptable to them. The method of "benchmarking" and dispute resolution are the primary areas of disagreement. As surgeons we want to help our patients have access to good care but the outcome of the discussion may cause financial difficulties for physicians and patients. It is important that physicians' voices are heard in the conversation.

2. Narrow networks are a related problem, and are frequently the cause of the surprise bill. However, narrow networks are a separate problem in their own right when insurance companies limit the options that their beneficiaries have to access necessary care. Provider directories are frequently out of date, and physicians may be unaware that they have been excluded from a network.

3. Physician ownership of ancillaries is important to many hand surgeons, primarily because physicians are in the best position to direct patient care. Physicians can often provide quality care in a less expensive and more efficient way than hospitals. Communication is better when physicians, therapists, and surgical and imaging facilities seamlessly share information. There are powerful voices on Capitol Hill who believe that there is an inherent conflict for physicians when they own the facilities where their patients receive care. These ownership arrangements are tightly regulated and are allowed currently as part of the group practice exception in the Stark law.

4. Requiring prior authorization for surgical procedures, advanced imaging studies, and many medications is common practice by insurance companies. These hurdles to patient care result in large amounts of wasted staff time and delays in timely care. Most of the time approval is given, which begs the question of who benefits from this process. There is currently a bill in Congress dealing with prior authorization.

5. Opioids, and the opioid epidemic have an impact on hand surgery practices. Regulations aimed at curbing excess prescribing and consumption are barriers to prescribing for acute situations, such as trauma or surgery. Also, these regulations can make it difficult for patients with long-term, stable opioid use to obtain their medications.

6. High prescription drug prices and high insurance policy deductibles have a combined detrimental effect on patients, often causing them to delay care or choose less expensive and possibly less efficacious treatments.

State issues affecting hand surgeons:

1. Scope-of-practice issues are perennial in most state legislatures. Many midlevel practitioners and other nonphysicians are trying to gain access to independent practice without going through the extensive training that physicians complete before they can practice. Team-based care is important in health care delivery and advocacy at the state level by physicians is important for our patients.

2. Workers compensation is a big part of hand surgery practice for many American Society for Surgery of the Hand (ASSH) members, because hand injuries are common in work settings. There is a broad range of regulations and laws that vary greatly by state that makes workers compensation a healthy part of the health care system in some states and a dysfunctional construct in others. Involvement in the political process can make a big difference at the state level because of the many different stakeholders in workers compensation.

3. Certificate of need laws exist in many states and represent a layer of regulation that seeks to control health care facilities (surgery centers and advanced imaging in particular). This type of market control has winners and losers and frequently results in restricted competition. Many states grapple with this issue on an annual basis.

These are but a few examples of the massive impact that legislatures at the federal and state levels can have on individual surgeons and health care systems. Patients are affected and it is our job to look out for them. This is done in several ways. ASSH recognizes the importance of advocacy and is constantly working to maximize the impact that surgeons can have on behalf of patients.

Currently, hand surgeons are represented in several different organizations via liaisons or direct representation. This includes the American Academy of Orthopedic Surgeons with their Orthopedic

PAC, the American College of Surgeons, the AMA, and the American Society of Plastic Surgeons. Our interests are most often in alignment with the other organizations representing the House of Medicine, especially those representing our surgical colleagues. The ASSH has previously looked at forming its own political action committee or hiring its own lobbyist but until now our representation has been through other organizations. Another avenue that is currently useful is advocacy by individual surgeons to their elected officials.

Developing a hand-specific advocacy program has strengths and weaknesses. Our society certainly has a deep understanding of the issues that affect hand surgeons. ASSH also has a long history of being a nimble and forward-thinking organization. However, our small size limits us in fundraising and also impact in comparison with other larger health care organizations. Hand surgery's multiple specialty makeup is a strength in broadening our reach but also a weakness because it dilutes our influence within other specialty organizations.

ASSH will continue to use its relationships with other organizations to strengthen the hand surgery agenda in Washington and in the states. Individual surgeon relationships with elected officials are extremely important and make a difference at all levels. ASSH may choose a different path to advocate for its members in the future but rest assured that everyone in leadership in our society understands the importance of representing hand surgeons in Washington and at the state level. In the meantime, here are some suggestions to help surgeons who are interested in developing their own advocacy skills.

AS INDIVIDUALS

Physicians are in a unique position to communicate with legislators and regulators. We address the nuts and bolts and communication skills next, but we must make an effort to engage. Most legislators have open houses at their district offices. They are interested in hearing from their constituents during those times, and the open house provides a good place to start building a relationship with the legislator and their staff. There does not need to be a pressing issue to underpin the visit. In fact, to start, it is probably better if there is not one. That allows for getting to know one another and perhaps identifying areas of mutual interest. Based on this relationship, you might become a "key contact" for your specialty organization. We will talk about this a bit more next.

There are opportunities for physicians, our staffs, and our families to get involved in campaigns, which is also an effective way to engage. Go to a fundraiser or make a contribution. Volunteer on a campaign, stuff envelopes, make some telephone calls, host a fundraiser. State medical and professional society advocacy staffs are helpful in facilitating and suggesting ways to get involved.

When a pressing issue does present itself, there are several ways to get involved. Direct advocacy is important, particularly if there is an established relationship. Write a letter or email. This is particularly effective if you know the staff person in charge of the area of concern. You may be contacted by a state or national association to weigh in on an issue, and there is frequently a hyperlink in the email that makes it simple to add your voice via email or a telephone call. There may be a public call for comment by a regulator. This is an opportunity for you to explain how the proposed rule might affect you or your patients in the real world.

We also have voices within our communities that we can use. Local newspapers frequently publish a letter to the editor, or an op-ed. Local media call-in shows are effective forums.

AS ORGANIZATIONS

Our professional societies can speak with the gravitas of representing all of us, in our specialty, or in our profession. That voice carries a significant weight in the discourse about medical and social matters. The professional and advocacy staff of these organizations have long-term relationships with all three branches of government, and sometimes serve as partners in developing and implementing policy. Many organizations and their staff have deep expertise in some medical and policy areas and serve as resources to legislators and regulators. That expertise is sometimes deployed via amicus curae briefs submitted to courts in support of policy positions, or in testimony to legislative committees.

AS INDIVIDUALS THROUGH ORGANIZATIONS

Advocacy by organizations is predicated on the policies adopted by those organizations. The process by which those policies are adopted varies. In specialty societies (American Academy of Orthopedic Surgeons, American Society of Plastic Surgeons, ASSH, AAHS, American College of Surgeons) this tends to occur through leadership, perhaps with validation by the general membership. In medical societies (AMA, State medical associations) this is more often via a deliberative process by a representative body, such as the AMA House of Delegates. Individuals can impact that policy by being active in these organizations.

Organizations mobilize their memberships for targeted issues. In addition to email and telephone campaigns, organizations also organize political action committees to leverage political contributions of the membership. Individuals can amplify their impact by contributing to a political action committee.

Many associations develop information materials and packets addressing a particular issue. They make those materials available to members identified as key contacts and ask them to deliver the materials to legislators.

Here are some specific important take-home messages for hand surgeons on successful advocacy:

1. Advocacy and the associated costs are part of a successful business model. Our situation as physicians could have been even more challenging but for the representation that we have with our advocacy groups and the physicians who do this work on behalf of all physicians. Join your professional societies. At the federal level the advocacy groups do much of the work and they frequently organize "fly in" opportunities to meet with legislators on Capitol Hill.

2. Personal relationships with legislators are important. It is easy to find your legislators at openstates.org and they look forward to hearing from constituents, especially people that they recognize. This is easier at the state level and relationships are easier to build when the legislator is not in session because of time constraints. Communication from a person known to the elected official is effective, especially a thoughtful email or a personal telephone call.

3. Follow political issues that affect your practice. Read your organizations' newsletters. Vote in every election. Frame all your communication with the impact on patients. We all are leaders in our work and our communities and we have a great opportunity to impact the political process.

Please contact either of us with any specific questions. We have a responsibility to protect our patients and our profession.

DISCLOSURE

The authors have nothing to disclose.

Moving?

Make sure your subscription moves with you!

To notify us of your new address, find your **Clinics Account Number** (located on your mailing label above your name), and contact customer service at:

Email: journalscustomerservice-usa@elsevier.com

800-654-2452 (subscribers in the U.S. & Canada)
314-447-8871 (subscribers outside of the U.S. & Canada)

Fax number: 314-447-8029

Elsevier Health Sciences Division
Subscription Customer Service
3251 Riverport Lane
Maryland Heights, MO 63043

*To ensure uninterrupted delivery of your subscription, please notify us at least 4 weeks in advance of move.

Printed and bound by CPI Group (UK) Ltd, Croydon, CR0 4YY

03/10/2024

01040307-0017